Praise for *Natural Childbirth Exercises*

No one knows more about Dr. Bradley's Husband-Coached Childbirth than Rhondda Hartman. As I worked side-by-side in his office with my beloved step-father, Dr. Robert Bradley, the amazing effect Rhondda had on our patients was proven daily with the successful outcomes of thousands of births. Get *Natural Childbirth Exercises*—for yourself and any one you know who is pregnant.

Susan Lindemann Nelson

With great enthusiasm, I highly commend the exercises and teachings of Rhondda Hartman. Does it make a difference? Indeed! Not only did I work closely with her, I delivered four of Rhondda's children (or as Dr. Bradley said, "caught") and know that what she recommends will benefit all pregnant women. *Natural Childbirth Exercises* is long overdue.

Max D. Bartlett, MD
Retired and former partner of Robert A. Bradley, MD

Rhondda's book is wonderful. I am so impressed with the way she shares her beautiful attitude about birth. I look forward to having *Natural Childbirth Exercises* become a warm, inspiring compliment to the Bradley Method Classes.

Marjie Hathaway, American Academy of
Husband-Coached Childbirth, Co-Founder of the
Bradley Method®

D1091648

Every pregnant woman needs this book. Rhondda's advice on birth and breastfeeding is pertinent and reliable. She knows childbirth first-hand as the mother of five and developer of childbirth exercises—she successfully accomplished what she writes about. Not only did she teach natural childbirth, Rhondda was a La Leche League leader and together, we started the League in Colorado.

Get *Natural Childbirth Exercises*—if you are a healthcare provider; if you are a partner or spouse of a pregnant woman; or if you are pregnant. Any and all will benefit from learning about and using these exercises that will ease the birth for both baby and mother.

Mary Ann Kerwin
Co-Founder of La Leche League International

Rhondda's classes and exercises prepared me beautifully for my son's birth. Her relaxing techniques really work! Read this book, practice her exercises, use her wisdom. It is all there in *Natural Childbirth Exercises*.

Roberta Scaer, co-author
Good Birth, Safe Birth

What a joy it was to work on *Natural Childbirth Exercises* with Rhondda Hartman. As a mother of four children, all natural childbirths, I wished I had had her as my guiding spirit as my belly grew and births approached. If I had only known about Rhondda, my pregnancies, my body and my births would have enjoyed full harmony!

Judith Briles
*Author YOU: Creating and Building the Author
and Book Platforms*

Natural Childbirth Exercises

for the Best Birth Ever

Exercises used by the Bradley Method®

Rhondda Evans Hartman

To Laura, with love, maternally, Rhondda E. Hartman 10/30/13

Natural Childbirth Exercises for the Best Birth Ever
Exercises used by the Bradley Method®
by Rhondda Evans Hartman

© 2013 by Rhondda Evans Hartman. All rights reserved. No part of this book may be reproduced in any written, electronic, recording, or photocopying without written permission of the publisher or author. The exception would be in the case of brief quotations embodied in the critical articles or reviews and pages where permission is specifically granted by the publisher or author.

Although every precaution has been taken to verify the accuracy of the information contained herein, the author and publisher assume no responsibility for any errors or omissions. No liability is assumed for damages that may result from the use of information contained within. The Bradley Method® and American Academy of Husband-Coached Childbirth® have been registered in the United States Patent Office. Only those teachers currently affiliated (as listed on *www.BradleyBirth.com*) with the American Academy of Husband-Coached Childbirth® may teach The Bradley Method®. For additional childbirth information contact: The Bradley Method®, Box 5224, Sherman Oaks, California, 91423-5224, USA or go to *www.BradleyBirth.com*.

Books may be purchased in bulk or otherwise, by contacting the publisher and author at: *MileHighPress@aol.com*

MileHigh Press

Mile High Press, Ltd.
PO Box 460880
Aurora, CO 80046

Cover and Interior Design: Nick Zelinger (NZ Graphics)
Editor: John Maling (Editing By John)
Creative Consultant: Judith Briles, (The Book Shepherd)

Library of Congress Catalog Number: 22013932902
ISBN: 978-1-885331-47-2 (print book)
ISBN: 978-1-885331-48-9 (e-book)

1) Childbirth   2) Pregnancy   3) Exercise   4) Women's Health

First Edition Printed in the United States

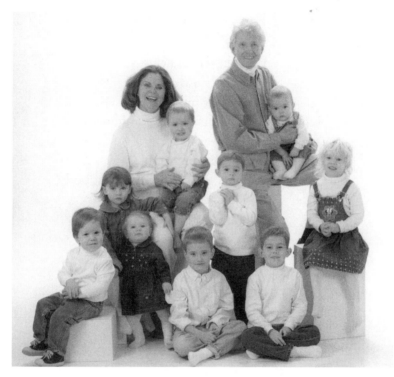

Dedicated to My Family with Love,
especially to the grandchildren for whom this book is intended:
Ford, Jon, Rienne, Rhys, Lillian, Austin, Reed, Ashby and Hart

Loose and Limp ... Warm and Heavy

Let your whole being
sink slowly, slowly, slowly.
Feel your muscles
becoming limp and loose and comfortable
Drifting or floating,
relaxed and comfortable,
warmth and heaviness spread through your body.
The baby in your uterus
is warm and heavy.
Feel warmth and heaviness
spreading from the baby to your abdomen, hips,
thighs, knees, lower legs, ankles,
feet, and toes.
Slowly, the lower half of you is
loose and limp,
warm and heavy.

The upper half of you awaits its turn.
Slowly release, let go,
warm and heavy,
limp and loose.
Let every cell absorb and enjoy,

spreading up back and front,
chest and shoulders.
Arms and fingers let go.

As your neck releases tension,
your head slowly shifts and becomes
more and more relaxed.
Nearer and nearer that comfortable state of
relaxation.

Erase the worries from your brow,
eyes loose but closed.
Eyes and all around eyes
limp and loose.
Cheeks loosen and droop,
jaw drops.
Tongue is loose in your mouth,
lips part slightly.
Warm, heavy, and comfortable.
Deep, slow, heavy breathing.
Breathe in and out slowly,
abdomen up and down slowly.
Limp and loose,
warm and heavy,
comfortably relaxed.

In your mind's eye
hold a softly purring kitten in your lap
while sunshine warms you both.

Listen to the laughter of children
sledding on a crisp sparkly snowy hill.

Ride a bicycle on a lazy autumn afternoon,
hair blowing in the wind.

Sit before a roaring, snapping fire
with a crisp apple ready to eat.
Watch a robin build her nest,
weaving string and straw with precision.

Lie on the warm sand, you and your love,
while the waves roll up on the beach.

Limp and loose,
warm and heavy,
comfortably relaxed.

— Rhondda Hartman

TABLE OF CONTENTS

From Dr. Robert A. Bradley

I was honored when Dr. Bradley wrote the Foreword for my first book, Exercises for True Natural Childbirth. *With this all new edition, I felt that it was appropriate to share his insightful words with you. REH*

Instinct is defined as "the innate propensity that incites animals to the actions that are essential for their existence, preservation, and development."

Human beings, though animals by virtue of our classification as mammals, apparently lack this innate propensity. As a result, we do not instinctively conduct our actions and behavior along pathways that will lead to preservation. Rather, from ignoring the great natural laws that manifest themselves automatically in the behavior of the other species of mammals in the bearing of their young to maintain and preserve their kind, we are not preserving but are gradually destroying our species, and even the environment and planet on which we live.

One pathway—and I consider it the most vital of all pathways to be preserved—is being destroyed as we bungle via drugs the reproduction of our species. Even before we clean up our external environment, we must first and foremost clean up the bloodstreams of our pregnant women, preventing their pollution with poisons and chemicals. Internal ecology must precede external, for drugs taken by pregnant women and laboring mothers have proved to have deleterious effects on the brain and body functions of their offspring.

Years ago, while in specialty training for obstetrics and gynecology, I proposed this as a theoretical possibility and earnestly suggested that human mothers, lacking instinct, should be trained to conduct themselves similarly to the other female mammals so that drugs and medications would be unnecessary in the reproduction of human babies. I felt not only that these drugs were temporarily harmful to newborn babies, obvious at just a cursory glance, but also that a subtle depletion of brain function persists throughout the lifetime of the individual.

I pointed out that by drugging mothers we are giving twenty times too large a dose to their unborn babies, as the baby receives the full dose of drug through the placental connection with the mother. Sir William Osler once stated that the main feature that distinguishes humans from other animals is the desire to take drugs.

Rhondda Hartman is a highly experienced teacher of true Natural Childbirth as well as being the mother of five husband-coached, un-medicated babies. She is a pioneer leader in the dawning of a new era of drugless childbirth, appropriately called "Natural Childbirth." What she teaches in this book is an exact copy of the instinctual behavior of similar mammals.

In following through my pet theory that you can teach humans how to perform "birthing" as well as, say, swimming—both actions being adroitly performed without instruction by all other mammals—I ran across innumerable obstacles, all of which can be overcome by the parents-to-be who carefully follow Mrs. Hartman's directions.

The first obstacle to overcome is that although people are designed amazingly like four-legged mammals, someone taught us to walk erect! As a consequence of this erect posture, not only do humans have unique problems, such as varicose veins on our "hind" legs, low backaches, toxemia of pregnancy, etc.—all of which are unheard of in our fellow mammals—but women's daily activities stiffen and weaken the muscles used in bearing babies.

The need for prenatal exercises to condition the childbearing muscles is obvious. I was delighted to have pointed out to me recently by an authority on whales and dolphins that these aquatic mammals go through a set pattern of daily prenatal exercises as soon as the female becomes pregnant, to strengthen their birth-giving muscles for later use.

Although it is fashionable now to assert that there is no difference between a man and a woman, I found this to be untrue in the demonstration of prenatal exercises. I needed women teachers to prepare women and Mrs. Hartman was one of the first to volunteer as a childbirth educator. She is not only a good teacher but is herself a shining example of what she teaches. In spite of her having borne five term babies, her body, as you can tell by the illustrations in this book, is beautiful, her posture perfect, and she can join her grown children in ballet and modern dance performances. On a visit to Russia as a Natural Childbirth educator, she encountered skepticism that such a slim, lithe body had given birth to five babies. How does she maintain her good figure? She tells us in this book. To any pregnant woman I would say, "Do thou likewise."

Mrs. Hartman not only prepares the bodies of pregnant women, but because of her personal experiences so generously shared, she further prepares the minds and souls of expectant mothers for the *joy* of childbirth.

As a former Officer and Director who currently serves on The Advisory Board of the American Academy of Husband-Coached Childbirth®, she helps train childbirth educators in the "Bradley Method®" of true Natural Childbirth. The film of four births available from the academy is appropriately labeled "Childbirth for the Joy of It," for with proper preparation human "animals" can enjoy spontaneous, un-medicated births.

Many young women refuse to walk in the outmoded pathways of yesterday. They want their babies to be born without drugs, and they want to share the joyful experience of natural birth with their husbands. Woe be to any doctor who has the reputation of being a "drugger"—who administers medication routinely to unprepared patients. Woe be to any hospital so backward as to still be clinging to outmoded rules.

The hope of a clean planet lies in the birthing without medication of intelligent, clear-brained babies who will grow up to solve our ecological problems. Not *more* babies but *better* babies result from following the example and teaching of this author, a true leader of new and better generations. Let's get back to nature, obstetrically, before it is too late.

Robert A. Bradley, A.B., M.D. (1917-1998)
Founder, American Academy of Husband-Coached Childbirth®

From Marjie Hathaway, AAHCC, The Bradley Method®

One of the primary principles of The Bradley Method and the Academy of Husband Coached Childbirth has always been exercise. Not just exercise, but exercise for true Natural Childbirth. Rhondda's first book, *Exercises for True Natural Childbirth* has been out of print for a number of years and has been missed. Now she has solved that problem with her new book, *Natural Childbirth Exercises for the Best Birth Ever: Exercises Used by The Bradley Method®*!

It details the exercises that Rhondda and Dr. Robert A. Bradley, both pioneers in the Natural Childbirth Movement, developed and used in his practice. These same exercises have been used by couples with The Bradley Method for nearly one million successful natural births.

Rhondda shares stories, the importance of a positive attitude about childbirth, explains and shows how to correctly do the exercises outlined and gives the reasoning behind them. She dispels the fear often associated with childbirth and gives women the confidence that they can give birth naturally. And she explains the effectiveness of physical preparation in an easy-to-understand manner. All of these ideas and procedures are very much needed today to offer an important alternative to popular, mainstream childbirth practices.

Rhondda's basic exercises remain classic and true to the needs of the pregnant female body. They remain essentially the same over the four decades of successful use in The Bradley Method classes.

Remember that childbirth is an athletic event! To bring home the gold ... these simple exercises need to be used, practiced and coached so that the mother and baby are ready for the most rewarding moment of their lives.

As a mother of five natural births, Rhondda is an expert and a beautiful example of The Bradley Method experience. She is an Advisor to the Academy, has supported The Bradley Method since its inception, and is a regular guest at our teacher trainings.

Natural Childbirth Exercises for the Best Birth Ever: Exercises Used by The Bradley Method® will be an important supplement to couples looking for a *how-to* for these exercises, as well as providing positive guidelines and examples while attending The Bradley Method classes. You will want to review it over and over again during your preparation for the Big Event!

> Marjie Hathaway, AAHCC, co-author of *Husband Coached Childbirth*
> by Dr. Robert A. Bradley; co-founder of The Bradley Method®
> and American Academy of Husband Coached Childbirth

How to Use This Book

N*atural Childbirth Exercises* will teach you, the reader, as though you are in a class with me. Within, you will find my total class instruction on paper so that you will know how to prepare for your labor. *My approach is strictly nonmedical and practical.* I intend to tell you how it feels to be pregnant and to give birth. In other words, my personal goal is to prepare your body, mind and spirit for this amazing event you are going through which will change your life.

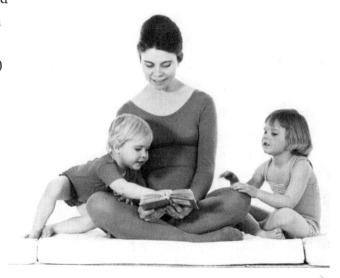

I am a mother of five, and cheerleader for over 14,000 mothers and their babies that attended my classes, not to mention the countless numbers who have read my other book, *Exercises for True Natural Childbirth*. I am a pioneer in the Natural Childbirth Movement and I developed the exercises with Dr. Bradley. I am very confident that if you will use the exercises recommended and described and do all the practicing that I tell you to do, you can enjoy your births. I did it and you can, too!

Dr. Bradley and I planned our education of Natural Childbirth as a joint effort for his Medical Obstetric Practice. He gave lectures to the couples to instruct them in the medical aspects of *Husband Coached Childbirth* and I taught the pregnant moms-to-be to prepare themselves mentally, physically and emotionally for the birth. I am convinced that everything I taught then is just as valid now as it was then. I believe that it is important that young women of today accept the responsibility of their own bodies, health and especially their own birth. No one can do it for you. You are the expert. You can do it. The rewards are stupendous.

As I write, I feel as though I know you. So this is a very personal experience between us … you and me. Teaching has been the greatest joy of my working career, but writing it, instead of saying it, has turned out to be the hardest, longest "labor" I've ever had.

I suggest you read the whole book quickly and then use it very methodically, exercise by exercise, so that you will really have your body and muscles ready by full-term pregnancy. I have developed the sequence of preparation based on my own experiences and the thousands of women I've worked with. Some of the basic, important postures you need to learn as soon as possible, which may be in your second or third month of pregnancy. Give yourself enough time to be really prepared by the time you have your baby. Do not wait until the last few weeks! In addition, I offer you other exercises or postures or "tricks" when you may need some relief from that pressure in your pelvis as the baby gets bigger and heavier.

The discussion of labor itself is left until you are quite close to delivery—six to eight weeks prior to due date. I have discovered in myself a strange detachment from serious acceptance of the labor until I was really facing it. This seems a fairly common reaction. When it's time, study the discussion of labor, how it feels, and what to do. Before this, it is a theory that most of us slip into the back of our minds—knowing it will happen. Just not today. In those last few weeks, you begin to deal with it as fact. The specific details of labor will make more sense to you later in pregnancy, when you are ready to accept the very hard work that having a baby requires. Labor is not easy but it is probably going to be the most wonderful work you will ever do.

Although you might want to gloss over the actual labor emotionally, you will need to be learning the physical techniques to get ready for it. That is the reason I teach relaxation and abdominal breathing at the beginning of *Natural Childbirth Exercises* but actually talk about labor and how it feels toward the end.

Today, most women still give birth at hospitals. That is what I have experienced and it is what I know and I will reference that. Many women choose other options—birth centers or home birth. I was one of a group who started a Birth Center in the pioneer days of Natural Childbirth. I have attended several home births. There is nothing more beautiful and exciting. There could be no more pleasant setting for a birth than in your own home, but that is not my expertise. I do know that wherever you give birth, the exercises that you will learn in this book will greatly enhance your experience for you and your baby.

I was trained as a Registered Nurse and that is what I know. I am also a Natural Childbirth Educator and know what it takes to have a successful natural birth. I am part of The Bradley Method and am on the Advisory Board of the American Academy of Husband Coached Childbirth. I highly recommend the Bradley Method and will reference it often in these pages.

If you plan to have a *home birth*, everything in this book is essential to you. Your physical and mental preparation is necessary no matter where you plan to give birth. I have tried to give you information that will be helpful as you plan for your choice of venue.

If you plan to have a *hospital birth*, begin early to find out what is offered to make your birth more like a home birth. Ask for the procedures to be changed to accommodate your ideal *birth plan*. Do not be timid. Ask for what you want. Hospitals are making every effort to create a homelike atmosphere in the birthing room, where you will be in one room for the whole of your birth experience from the time you are admitted to the time you leave for home with your baby in your arms.

Attending a Bradley Method class in your community will be the perfect complement to this book. The information given by a Bradley Method Teacher will fit nicely with the information in this book. Become familiar with the Bradley website—*www.BradleyBirth.com*. You will discover that it has a state-by-state map that identifies instructors, there may be one just down the street from you.

In these classes, local information is shared that will help you in your choices of Health Care Professionals, hospitals, birth options, and a myriad of other opportunities. Your teacher will be answering questions you did not know to ask. You will also make friends. It's not uncommon that get-togethers continue post-birth as a "new mom community". After all, there is a shared experience.

If you cannot find a Bradley Class for your "method" of Natural Childbirth close by, pick one and learn what you can from it. Do not accept that a medicated birth is the only option! Your local hospital most likely has classes and/or support groups. The Internet becomes an ally. Search for "Natural Childbirth classes" and see what pops up. At my last checking, I found over 139,000 entrees! When you narrow the search to your specific city, the number will drop dramatically, a number that you can easily track.

Read everything you can during early pregnancy, and then choose the method or theory and a teacher who most appeals to you. Look for truly non-medicated Natural Childbirth, which describes the harmful results of medications for the mother and baby. Once you are committed to a class, make sure the philosophy is true Natural Childbirth. What the Bradley Method offers is the most basic, most practical method there is—one of the primary reasons for its success. There will be easy, effective techniques and loads of information taught; along with research to make you understand why you want *no medications*. There will be discussions regarding the procedures which may be common but are not necessary when you and your baby are unmedicated. You need to find a Bradley Method Teacher and class.

Throughout, I've made references to other books which I hope you'll read. There are many, many good books on the detailed physiology of childbirth, and for that reason I have limited myself to the subjective preparation and sensations of having a baby. Rather than what is happening medically during childbirth, I've stressed how it feels. However, I've tried to answer "why" as well. My hope is that I've answered your need. May you have a healthy and happy pregnancy and a joyful childbirth! Check my website, *www.NaturalChildbirthExercises.com* for more references, book reviews and birth related discussions.

I have not dealt with complications, it's not my expertise—that is what the doctor is trained to do. In these pages, I refer only to the normal, uncomplicated pregnancy. It is a *fact* that at least 90 percent of you can have your babies absolutely naturally with no analgesia or anesthesia prior to the birth. In Dr. Bradley's records, 3 percent of the total required Caesarean sections knew from the beginning, that medically they could not have a natural birth. They took the classes anyway and went into labor before the surgery. Of the remaining 97 percent, 3.6 percent had unforeseen complications, and 93.4 percent achieved spontaneous, uncomplicated, un-anesthetized births—an amazing statistic. The National Vital Statistics System reported that in The United States in 2007, Caesareans represented 32 percent of all births. How times have changed!

You can be successful by doing your part as well as you can. Relax and work with your body. Even if a complication should occur, you will have done your relaxing and helped the uterus to do its job. There are usually many hours in a labor, even if anesthesia becomes necessary, all your training will be very helpful. The exercises are your guide to a healthy, strong body for your lifetime.

In other words, Natural Childbirth training will be helpful to all, even if you happen to be one who needs medical intervention. No matter what, your pregnancy will be more pleasant, with all this preparation.

If you will use the exercises that have been developed by Dr. Bradley and me and described within *Natural Childbirth Exercises*, I am confident that your birthing experience will be a memorable, joyful and exciting one. Have I led you to believe that having a baby is easy? No. Please note, I did not say easy or even painless. Childbirth is work. Embrace the work. You cannot win any athletic event without hard work. When you are educated about the work you are undertaking and use the tools that I have given you to enhance it, you will be thrilled by the outcome just as my husband and I were with each of our five births.

My hope is that you will accept childbirth for what it is, labor. It is more work going on in your body than you've ever experienced. I hope you will appreciate the forces and be in awe of what is happening during the birth process. If you are well prepared, you will not let those forces overwhelm you, but will work with them to accomplish the goal.

These nine months are a great period in your life. Enjoy and experience them to the fullest.

Happy *birth* day!

Chapter 1

Congratulations ... Now You Are Pregnant!

As you begin your pregnancy it is very exciting and almost unreal. It is so ever-present in your mind that it's hard to believe it doesn't show to anyone you pass on the street.

+ You feel so new and different.
+ You think about new philosophies of life.
+ You become aware of the environment around you as totally changed.
+ You find yourself communicating with the wee one that is growing within you.
+ You find yourself gently caressing your tummy.

Some of the newness and change is somewhat unpleasant. Things bother you that have never bothered you before—the creak of the bathroom door can be screamingly irritating. Your husband's unexpected love pat makes you cry. ("It hurt," you say, wondering why you are crying.) You feel "left out" at work when you are not invited to join a group for lunch, a group that you never wanted to join in the past.

You find that your pending "mommyhood" has introduced a new vocabulary, one that used to amuse you when others used it. You discover things about your body that you never knew—where did those breasts come from—and those cravings—and your reaction to certain smells? And yes, you silently enjoy that tenderness you feel toward your spouse/partner in the creation of what will be in your arms within a few months.

Are you nodding your head? Do you know what I'm saying? Perhaps you were the rare exception and escaped this normal but weird experience of early pregnancy. I have to tell you, I was shocked when I first became pregnant. Newly married for two months, I didn't envision nor want a baby so early in our relationship. My husband, Richard, was just fine with it. I had to get my head around it … after all … I had only known and loved the man for three months!

Welcome to the wide-world of hormonal changes during pregnancy.

You have so many things to think about with this new situation in your life called pregnancy. Suddenly you are faced with all sorts of new things. What should you eat to be sure the baby is healthy? What changes will have to be made in your home? Will you have to move? Perhaps a two-year-old has to be moved out of a crib. How will you make your wardrobe accommodate your expanding tummy? Will you have to quit your job? Can you manage on one salary? No matter what, your life will be changed forever.

By now you will have experienced the strange phenomena that your pregnancy creates in others. Everyone is an expert and has advice to offer. The mailman, the boss, the shoe salesperson, your parents, the woman next door, the grocery shopper behind you as you checkout at the supermarket. They all have tales to tell. Reactions vary from "How lovely" to "Poor little thing," or even, "There are enough children in the world already."

You collect old wives' tales and folk medicine everywhere you go. You'll get some good advice, too, but sorting it all out is the problem.

In the Beginning

You will have days of elation and excitement and you will have bad days. You may even have day-after-day of nausea or (I hope not) of vomiting. I will talk more on this subject later. Ideally, you and your husband or partner can maintain good communication throughout this time in your pregnancy. It's vital to you both. Never have you needed a sounding board more, and never has your need for reassurance been greater.

You are normal and healthy and want to have this baby. Say so. A close, loving relationship is so important to the role of parenting. Sharing your love for each other with your baby increases the amount of love, it does not decrease it. It will enrich your life. It will make the relationship with each other bigger and wider as you expand to include another family member. But you are not sure of that yet and it's okay to be a bit worried about sharing your life with another person. The worry will be gone when you hold your baby in your arms.

Your sex life may change, too. Your spouse should know that he is not being punished or rewarded, depending on which direction your needs take. Talk with him about the changes in you. You may not get to understand yourself any better, but at least your spouse will learn that you don't know what's going on any more than he does. The most important thing for your relationship is to keep talking and listening to each other.

Stop and think of all the variations in your life because you conceived. Loosen up, relax, take a deep breath, and stop being so hard on yourself. Accept your pregnancy and allow yourself some limitations. Don't try to pretend that you are exactly the same person you were two or three months ago. You aren't.

At the same time, don't try to accept it all in one big swallow. It's always hard for the female; we have to accept motherhood in a matter of a week or two, whereas the father can take nine months to grasp his role. Every one of us has gone through the whole gamut of emotions. We each do it our own way.

Now let's get back to that initial response to your pregnant state—excitement! That seems to be the prevailing and overriding emotion that surpasses all the other reactions and keeps you going.

I am making the assumption that since you are reading *Natural Childbirth Exercises*, you are interested in experiencing *Natural Childbirth*. That's wonderful news.

What is Natural Childbirth?

+ Natural Childbirth is, well, natural.

+ Natural Childbirth is having a baby without drugs.

+ Natural Childbirth is taking responsibility for your childbirth experience.

+ Natural Childbirth is preparing your body for an athletic event called Birth.

+ Natural Childbirth is having this baby the way you want even if it means going against cultural norms.

+ Natural Childbirth is making the decision that this is your body, your baby and no one knows better than you what is right for you during the 9 months of pregnancy and during the birth of your baby.

+ Natural Childbirth is a choice that you and your spouse/partner make and share together.

+ Natural Childbirth is a preparation of body, mind and spirit for giving birth and raising a child to become a successful adult.

+ Natural Childbirth is the most exciting, exhilarating, joyful, amazing event in your whole life. There is nothing that compares to it. Do not let anyone take this incredible life experience from you.

+ Natural Childbirth is accepting that you know what is best for you during your pregnancy and birth and that you are the expert. You will gladly take advice from the professionals but the decisions will be yours to make.

When you tell others that you plan on having "Natural Childbirth," you will encounter a variety of attitudes. Most of you already have firm ideas about how you want to have a baby but once you commit yourself to it, you will need to be able to defend what you are doing.

Many people will say, "You are so brave."

I am not brave enough to have a baby any other way! How can anyone be brave enough to give up total responsibility for the birth of her baby? Yet for years it was accepted practice that the doctor would, "Take care of you."

"Leave it all to me; I know what's best for you; trust me," was commonly heard when women gave birth prior to the 1950s.

It was a myth. It is still a myth. You are the one who knows what is best for you. You will need to have some teaching and skill-training because we have not been included or involved when our mothers and sisters and friends were giving birth. Do not count soley on instinct because our brains are better developed than that. We are able to learn from one another.

Natural Childbirth is a sharing of birth experiences with one another.

> No one can have your baby for you.
> No one but you can make it easy for you.
> Trust yourself and your body.
> Do this for the sake of your baby.
> Do this for yourself.

You must accept this as your responsibility. You *will* have this baby. You *will* prepare your body to give birth, and you *will* understand what is happening in your body to be able to work with the birth rather than against it.

Birth is a natural process. There is a natural opening in your body which allows the birth of the baby. Your body is designed for this process. You are not sick or ill or abnormal when pregnant. You are in a normal, natural, healthy state of pregnancy.

We enjoy a society that takes the precaution of hospital deliveries so that most of the complications associated with childbirth can be safely cared for by medical expertise. But that does not mean that you should be subjected to medical methods when you can give birth with joy, love, and lots of plain, honest hard work. It may even be easy, but don't count on that!

Explain, when you are asked, that we are using *educated* childbirth rather than *medicated* childbirth. You must prepare very carefully so that you will understand what your body is doing as you give birth and you will be able to work with the forces of birth. This makes for ease—not disease. Pregnancy and birth are not abnormal, unnatural, diseased states of your life, but rather, normal and natural—and we hope to add the ease.

The term, Natural Childbirth has many connotations in people's minds. You will get all types of reactions from people as you declare your intentions to have a natural birth.

Some consider it primitive—true Natural Childbirth is educated.

Some think it is an endurance test—true Bradley Natural Childbirth is good preparation.

Some think of it as training for the type of anesthesia your doctor will use—true Natural Childbirth uses absolutely no drugs or medication unless complications arise. When medication is necessary, you are in a medical situation. You are no longer in control of your birth.

Some think of it as a home delivery with no skilled medical person to "get in the way"—true Natural Childbirth is a birth with a health care provider who has good support from the whole medical community whether at home or in a birth center or in a hospital.

Some think it is not making use of the medical expertise that has been developed over the years—true Natural Childbirth is based on the newest scientific evidence that any anesthetic drug given prior to the birth of the baby does get into the baby's system, yes, even a local, and any dosage which will be effective for the mother is a huge overdose for her infant. How scary is that!

Some say that Natural Childbirth is unsafe—yet the very basis for Natural Childbirth is the decreased risk from anesthesia and unnecessary medical intervention for both mother and baby. It is the only safe way to protect the health of both. As a secondary benefit, it has turned out to be the most pleasant way to have a baby.

Some may say that Natural Childbirth causes great guilt and disappointment in those who do require anesthesia— true Natural Childbirth creates satisfied parents who did their best. Certainly it's disappointing to need a Caesarean section or to have some complication requiring the use of forceps and therefore, anesthesia, or to have your doctor prescribe an anesthetic for medical reasons. As long as each woman is consulted and included in the decision and given the medical reasoning that was used by the doctor, why would there be guilt?

A mother-to-be must be convinced that her doctor has her best interests in mind and that he did not "put one over on her." Then there is never a problem.

The burden is on the health care provider to use anesthesia only when necessary, to reassure the parents of the need for anesthesia when used, and to make sure the doctor has the complete trust of the parents. Surely that is not asking too much of our medical community!

Unfortunately, you will have to make sure that you do not choose a doctor who wants to use all the medical tools available. Some feel like they are a failure if *you* are able to have a natural birth with no drugs or medical intervention. Find a healthcare provider who supports *you*.

Natural Childbirth is a practical approach to having a baby which trains the woman and her partner for their roles in labor. The doctor supports the parents in labor and uses medical intervention only in those rare cases when it is necessary. All three work together as a team. The doctor is the lifeguard, the father or partner the coach, and the mother does the work!

Your First Big Decision

One of the biggest decisions you must make is to choose a healthcare professional that will be your guide, cheerleader and attendant for the birth of your baby. You want to choose one that wants for you the birth that you want to have. Interview at least three providers before selecting one. Whether you use a physician, midwife, or other healthcare provider, it will be your choice.

By the way, I will interchange the terms health care provider, midwife and doctor for ease of communicating with you throughout *Natural Childbirth Exercises*. Because I did have a doctor, it may be my most common term.

Interviewing a professional takes courage and a willingness to be comfortable to admit your lack of knowledge of the subject. You need to ask a lot of questions even when you think the questions are stupid. The way you are treated by the Health Care Provider will tell you a great deal about whether that is the right choice for you. This is a very important decision in your life and you do need to prepare carefully.

Questions you need to ask include:

+ What is the established routine of prenatal care?
+ What type of preparation for childbirth is offered?
+ What is the protocol regarding medications?
+ What type of support will be offered to you in labor?
+ Who will be expected and allowed to stay with you during your labor?
+ What is the attitude to your needs and wishes regarding the childbirth experience?
+ Has the professional had experience with Natural Childbirth?
+ Does he/she have any negativity toward this?

Your husband or partner can be of much help in making your desires known to the doctor and in assessing the situation. Be prepared with your idea of the perfect birth. Keep a list and discuss it together before you meet and interview your prospective health care provider. In most cases, you'll have a choice of health care providers, so do a bit of "shopping," then choose the one who best meets your expectations. If you have only one choice (such as living in a community with just one doctor who delivers babies), then proceed very slowly and cautiously, even deviously, to get your own way. One of my doctor friends told me that you must seduce to get your way, not attack. Know what you want and expect to get it but don't be abusive about it.

For help in techniques of interviewing your medical provider, you need to become educated yourself. It is one thing to ask dumb questions but quite another to actually choose not to find out the answers. Being pregnant and choosing to remain ignorant is not good for you or your baby. There are many ways of doing this. Much of it will be from reading everything you can. Read, read, and read! Talk to anyone who has had the experience of a natural birth. Check my website, *www.NaturalChildbirthExercises.com* for resources and references. I list books, websites and organizations that I consider helpful and will update them as needed.

All this adds up to the fact that you will have nine months of explaining what you plan to do in the name of Natural Childbirth. There may even be some large gaps in definition of Natural Childbirth between you and your doctor. Begin early to choose them so that your labor can be as relaxed as possible. Husbands/partners are essential in helping create good communication with your doctor. Ask positively, but do not demand, lest you nip all progress in the bud.

Getting on Schedule

Your health care provider will have a schedule of routine appointments for check-ups for you during your pregnancy. These are important. So little seems to be accomplished that you may have the urge to skip some but really, much information is recorded at these appointments. Small changes in you—especially in blood pressure, rapid weight gain and swelling—need to be noted so possible problems are prevented.

There are large volumes of statistics which prove the health and life of mothers and babies are vastly improved with good prenatal care. Allow the medical professionals to use their skill in preventing problems that will complicate your pregnancy. Do this for your baby's wellbeing and your own.

Let me add a word about asking your very busy doctor/midwife questions. I have found it helpful if I have a businesslike list of questions for my visit to the health care provider's office. It will facilitate things for all of you. Don't overdo and have three pages full. Write down the responses you get, it's easy to forget once you leave the office. The doctor knows your problems have been answered and you go home with a good feeling of satisfaction. Build a friendly but serious relationship with your doctor. If you can't manage that, then you are working with the wrong professional. Look for and hire another.

Old wives' tales can be a bother at this time of early pregnancy because with all that unsolicited advice you are getting, you don't know what to believe. Here are a few examples:

"Never raise your hands over your head."

"You mustn't hold in your tummy."

"If your nose grows, you're going to have a girl."

"If you have morning sickness, you're going to have a boy."

"If you have heartburn, the baby will have lots of hair."

"If you feel ugly and awkward, you'll have a girl."

"If you feel pretty, you'll have a boy."

"If the hair on your legs grows more slowly in pregnancy, it's a girl."

The list is endless ... and ridiculous!

If you feel troubled about whether or not they are nonsense, do ask your doctor. Remember, we are not very far out of the Victorian era when pregnant females did not even go out in public. Imagine the angst today's pregnant woman would have created in those times with her baby-bump openly displayed in form-fitting clothes or wearing a bikini.

Some old wives' tales are based on shreds of outdated fact, but most of them you can ignore—especially all the ones I've listed above.

Rhondda's Tip

The wise mom-to-be will surround herself with people and information about Natural Childbirth. Dismiss old wives' tales and explore in your community where Affiliated Bradley Method® instructors offer classes. You can find them by going to *www.BradleyBirth.com* or searching the internet for Bradley Method instructors in your city.

Chapter 2

Exercises for the First Trimester ... Tailor Sit

By the time you are three months pregnant, your baby weighs about one ounce. The baby has definitely become a boy or a girl, but you may not want to know. Arms and legs begin to move. The head is developed, with eyes, ears, nose and mouth. The bones have begun to form in that tiny body. The whole sac in which the baby grows is about the size of a goose egg.

Exercises for the First Trimester

Exercises do not have to be calisthenics. In most cases, *Natural Childbirth Exercises* are postures and not exercises at all—but exercise is an easy word to use. Many of the exercises that I developed were in collaboration with Dr. Robert Bradley, author of *Husband Coached Childbirth*. These exercises concentrated on your posture and your daily activities. Do not expect to break into a sweat—think of this as a very relaxed form of exercise which helps strengthen your body for pregnancy and giving birth.

The goal is to get your body into shape—you do not compete with anyone—you do the best *you* can. Most of our postures are designed to be used around the home in your everyday activities. Many can be done anywhere you work, but all can easily be fit in if you work at house all day. Some are to be used for your pregnancy and some prepare you for labor. However, many are to be maintained for the rest of your life.

Do not make yourself stiff and sore by overusing your muscles at first. Begin slowly and increase gradually and you will have pleasant results. You will be the judge of how many times you should do each posture. I'll give you guidelines in many cases—but remember that you are the one who will have the baby.

If your muscles are not ready for labor, who is to blame?

Some of the exercises and techniques you will be learning will be for labor but must be learned now and practiced throughout your pregnancy so that you will be good at it when you are in labor. For example, if you haven't practiced enough on your abdominal breathing, it's very hard to learn while in labor. Enlist the help of your husband or your labor coach to remind you. Get a good nine months of training. It will be to your benefit if you are diligent.

Let's begin with our first "exercise"—tailor sitting.

Tailor Sit

Never stand when you can sit; and when you sit—tailor sit!

Why?

Because tailor sitting is comfortable. Children and more "natural" cultures use this position without teaching.

Sitting tailor fashion, with your elbows on your knees, tilts the heavy uterus forward, away from your back and up and out of the pelvis. This teeter-totter effect, with the uterus tilted over the front of the pelvic bone, allows release of pressure and therefore permits good circulation of blood to the pelvic area, to kidneys, vagina and legs. The blood carries nutrients and oxygen to the uterus and your baby.

Tailor sitting keeps you from sitting in a chair in the usual manner—leaning back and allowing a backward tilt of the uterus—which puts pressure on blood vessels supplying the kidneys, uterus and legs, thereby reducing circulation. Crossing your knees further aggravates the problem and reduces circulation to the vagina.

Tailor sitting stretches and makes flexible the muscles of your bottom and the inner aspects of your thighs, enabling you to put your legs farther apart in second-stage labor, which will be helpful.

It may sound ridiculous, but the effect of increased light and air to your perineum is a healthy extra as it will help prevent vaginal yeast infections.

HOW:

Sit on the floor or any firm surface. Cross your ankles and bring them close to your body with knees wide apart. You may lean back slightly to reduce the weight on your ankles. A small pillow under the tail bone will also reduce pressure and may be more comfortable. This is not an exercise but rather a posture.

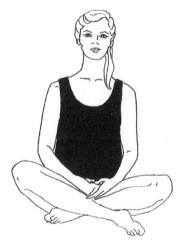
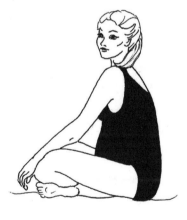

Variations: You may use variations to keep comfortable while sitting for longer periods. As one position becomes crampy, change to a variation:

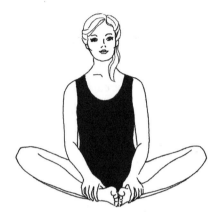

+ Soles of feet together, with knees bent and wide apart.

+ Stretch and move your feet and legs until you are comfortable.

+ Resume classic Tailor Sit.

Do not sit in any one position for long periods of time or your legs will go to sleep from lack of good circulation. Even if you sit in a chair, you don't punish yourself by never moving! Most of us find this tailor sitting position easy from all our activities in normal life but if it is difficult for you, rest your elbows on your knees with slight pressure. Do this for short periods. Never make yourself uncomfortable! Don't force your knees to the floor. That is not necessary and may be painful.

After a few weeks, you'll be comfortable for longer periods and your knees will come closer to the floor. Your knees may never touch the floor, since individuals differ. If you are very limber and your knees do touch the floor, this position will be very easy for you to use. You are ahead of most of us in preparation for Natural Childbirth!

There are problems other than muscles that can keep you from doing tailor sitting, I discovered. One evening when I was teaching a class to tailor sit, we had a guest who had come with her friend. She participated in the class with enthusiasm until I had explained the tailor sit position and asked everyone to use it. Our guest refused. She had been brought up in Mexico where young ladies conducted themselves in a formal way and sitting cross-legged on the floor—tailor sitting did not fit into her life style at all! I encouraged her, and I encourage you, to try the loose, easy, relaxed informality that suits our day and age and makes pregnancy so much easier.

WHERE:

Always choose a hard, level surface so that your hips and feet are on the same plane. Tucking a small pillow under your tail bone as you are getting used to this position may be more comfy but as you become good at it you will find a padded hard surface such as a carpeted floor much more to your liking.

WHEN:

Anytime you can sit down! For example:

+ Reading to the children or yourself, needlework, or whatever handicrafts you enjoy.

+ Cleaning drawers or lower cupboards (take the drawer out of the chest and put it on the floor).

+ Riding in a car, watching television, writing letters, watching movies, eating dinner at a coffee table or sitting on the floor—usually in your own home.

+ Playing cards or any games when you can sit on the floor instead of in a chair. Can't you see a foursome for bridge sitting on the floor practicing their tailor sitting?

+ During a conversation—sit on the floor, not on the sofa.

+ Folding clothes from the dryer.

+ With children, tailor sit for everything you do. You will be on their level as you diaper, dress, feed, cuddle, hug, listen, talk, play, fix a hurt, pick up toys—the list is twenty-four hours long!

+ You can sit this way in many chairs—from the ordinary hard kitchen chair (you may need a pad for your ankles) to one that is cushy and comfortable.

+ What other ways can you think of to use tailor sitting?

Sit in the tailor position for short periods or as long as it is comfortable. One woman told me in a class that she was having trouble with this posture. She claimed that it caused her legs to fall asleep. I checked her position and it was perfect. I reviewed some minor variations and she knew them all. But she insisted that it was still very uncomfortable for her to sit in the tailor position. We talked about where and when she was sitting this way and it all sounded normal.

Since tailor sitting is an uncomplicated position, there had to be a reason for her discomfort. I began to ask her a few questions. It seemed she was having the most trouble with her legs falling asleep during TV watching. I was ready to give up and tell her to keep trying and gradually her legs would become more used to it, when I had a flash thought. I had not asked how many minutes of TV she watched without moving.

Sure enough, her idea of a reasonable amount of time was not the amount that her legs could tolerate. She was sitting through a TV movie, two hours, without getting up and moving around. This is a superhuman effort when you are pregnant. Actually it is not good for you anytime!

My point is that you must use a certain amount of good sense in how you begin a new posture or exercise. Do it as often and as long as you like but do be kind to yourself and gradually work up to your optimum.

If tailor sitting is easy for you, it will be used for a more extended period of time than if you find it difficult. However, it should be used with the idea that you are not trying to set a new record. Make it a part of your life—a useful and comfortable addition to your way of doing things which will also contribute to your health. Think of tailor sitting as your *friend, not as an enemy.*

Rhondda's Tip

Everybody sits ... but how do you sit? Learning the Tailor Sit will ease the strain that many feel today with the extended sitting time that computer usage has created. It's smart to get up often and use your body ... but when you sit, Tailor Sit!

Chapter 3

Pelvic Rock ... with Variations

This exercise could be the most important addition to your wellbeing that you have ever learned! It is important to you now during your pregnancy and your birth but it is just as important for the rest of your life.

Dr. Bradley compares us to four footed animals in his *Husband Coached Childbirth* and so we imitate animals in Natural Childbirth. In the pelvic rock, we imitate four-footed animals in posture and it feels so good! As the uterus becomes heavier and heavier with pregnancy, standing upright causes it to push lower and more tightly into the pelvis. This compresses the blood vessels and interferes with circulation to the uterus, legs, and kidneys. The heavy uterus also stretches supportive ligaments that are attached in the small of the back at roughly the same position as in four-footed mammals.

The pressure and the weight cause the pregnant female to "give in" to the uterus, letting it fall forward and sway her back. Backache and pressure pains are the result. Pelvic rocking on hands and knees allows the uterus to fall forward, releasing the pressure in the pelvis and causing no discomfort in the spine because of the all-fours position. In this posture, your spine is a bridge supported on either end by arms and legs, whereas in a standing position your spine is an upright pole supporting you. A bridge can be sturdy with a sway in it, but get out of the way of a swaying pole!

The rule of Pelvic Rock is this:

When standing hold your spine straight so that the baby is contained in the pelvis. At regular intervals get on all-fours to do pelvic rocks for the release of pressure in your pelvis. Allowing the uterus to tip out of the pelvis improves circulation to the area but will cause back pain if you do it standing upright. That is why it is done on all fours!

Pelvic rock will strengthen and tone the muscles in the back and abdomen which will allow you to keep a straight spine and avoid back aches as the uterus pulls on the inside of your back. The uterus is attached by ligaments on the inside of your lower back so as it gets heavier with the baby's growth you need to have very strong muscles in your back along the spine to maintain good posture.

To recap: a straight back when standing with regular all fours pelvic rocks to release the uterus and let it hang out!

WHY?

What does pelvic rocking do for you? I will give you a long list of benefits, but the basic result is that you will be healthier and feel more comfortable. This is an exercise to help you during pregnancy. It strengthens muscles in your back and abdomen and therefore makes it easier for you to carry the baby in your pelvis. These muscles are also involved with the birthing process.

Pelvic rocking improves your posture for the rest of your life. This is a lifetime exercise. A straight spine makes you feel and look better whether you are pregnant or not. Pelvic rocking strengthens your back muscles.

The muscles along your spine need to be very strong to be able to maintain a straight spine while a heavy uterus is attached to it.

Pelvic rocking strengthens abdominal muscles to support the uterus, and what a difference that makes in your figure immediately after birth. Your tummy will be flatter than ever before. You may even reduce the size and flabbiness of your hips and thighs. You will no doubt be happy about your return to normal after the birth all because of this wonderful Pelvic Rock.

Pelvic rocking will help prevent varicose veins by increasing circulation to pelvis and legs. Relieving the pressure of the uterus in the pelvis will relieve pressure on the blood vessels. Any mild exercise improves circulation, so by pelvic rocking you are restoring good circulation to your pelvis and legs.

The relief of pelvic pressure and increased circulation helps prevent hemorrhoids, too.

Pelvic rocking increases mobility of the pelvis, which may help in labor as you push the baby through the birth canal.

Pelvic rocking will definitely help relieve tensions and relax you in preparation for bed at night.

Do extra when you are "too tired to do any."

HOW:

Get on the floor in an "all-fours" position, making sure that you form a Box position. Have your knees and hips in a line and your wrists and shoulders in a line, both of these 'lines' are perpendicular to the floor. Your knees may be comfortably apart.

1. Lower your abdomen toward the floor until you look like a "sway-back horse." But only so that you are comfortable. It may be a very small movement.

2. Lift your lower back until your back is parallel with the floor.

3. Tighten buttocks. This raises the back slightly and tightens the abdomen.

4. Slowly return to the "sway-back" position with control.

5. Repeat movements 2 through 4.

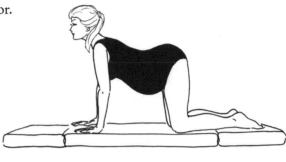

This must be done rhythmically, with as much control lowering as raising the back. It should be done slowly, the whole movement taking about five to seven seconds.

Do not move your shoulders and upper back. This exercise is for the lower back and pelvis and we ignore the upper back completely. It is a different exercise when you raise your upper back and is not specifically helpful in pregnancy or birth. Do it as a separate exercise if you want but I have not included it. Do not move your arms either.

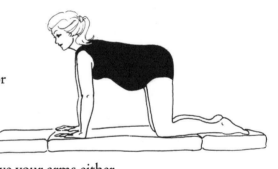

Watching yourself in a mirror while doing this exercise will help you do the movements. Instead of a full-length mirror, try putting a light on the floor to cast your shadow on the wall.

If you develop a pain or a "stitch" in your side as when running, it is a result of dropping your abdomen too quickly or too low. Stop and check to see how you are doing the movement. Be cautious with how low your back goes down. Sometime just tightening the back muscles is all you need to do. It does not have to be a large movement. Use more control and there will be only comfort, never discomfort.

WHERE:

It is very hard to combine this with any routine in your life unless you are beautifully uninhibited, as was my Natural Childbirth teacher, Peggy Rice. At a cocktail party one evening where everyone was rather formal, pregnant Peggy felt a nagging backache. She put her drink down and in her long dress, got on the floor on all fours and began pelvic rocking, chatting all the while to a very startled male guest.

If you can't emulate Peggy, you will have to get off by yourself several times during the day to do enough pelvic rocks to keep you comfortable. For those of you working outside your homes through a pregnancy, you might find a ladies' lounge or an unused conference room, a supply room—anyplace where you can get on all fours and do pelvic rocks to relieve the tension in your back. The first thing you should do as you walk into your home after work is to get down on your knees—double meaning intended! If your family is waiting impatiently for dinner, make it a routine to have some favorite snacks in the pantry for an appetizer so that you can take time to give your uterus and back some much needed relief.

WHEN:

Do the pelvic rock the last thing before bed—that is very important. Do 80 before bed, with a rest in the middle if you need it. Caution: do not start by doing this number. Work up gradually toward the goal of 80 before bed. Try 10 at a time to begin and make sure that you do not make your back stiff and sore by overworking these underused muscles!

Do at intervals during the day. For example: midmorning, midafternoon, and early evening, 40 each time (start with 10 and increase gradually), then 80 at bedtime. I suggest you increase to eighty when you are able to do so comfortably.

After your bedtime pelvic rocks, crawl into bed. Organize your body into the side lying Relaxation position discussed in the next chapter. Now your body is in the perfect posture for the comfort and health of baby and you. You are not lying on the baby nor is the baby's weight resting on you.

If this is your first pregnancy, you may not feel the need of the daytime pelvic rocks until your uterus has grown big enough to make you aware of a bit of pressure. Do them anyway. Start exercising those muscles! If you have already had a child, you'll want to pelvic rock all day long because it feels so good.

Rest position during pelvic rock

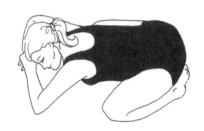

If your arms become tired before finishing the required eighty at bedtime, you may use this posture for a few minutes then continue with **pelvic** rocking. Dr. Bradley calls this the "froggy" position. Your back should be level with the floor. If your tail bone is sticking way up in the air, **do not use this position**. A "Knee-chest" position has a possibility of harm during pregnancy. But the "Pose of the Child" position or the Froggy is a very relaxing posture.

If you are not flexible enough to do this posture correctly then roll onto your side in a relax position to rest your arms before finishing your Pelvic Rocks before bed.

1. Kneel, spread knees a bit farther apart and have toes pointing straight back.

2. Sit back on your heels and then let your torso bend forward toward the floor so that your arms can rest on the floor and your head rests on your arms.

If this is not comfortable (you will need stretchy or very loose clothing), use a pillow under your chest and head ... or rest in a side relaxation position. This is a position meant to be used for your comfort so if it is not comfortable simply roll onto your side and relax in the side relax position. When your arms feel better get on all fours and resume Pelvic Rocks.

3. When you have finished your pelvic rocks, carefully get up and continue your activities or crawl into your bed for a good night of sleep.

Variations of Pelvic Rock

Since Pelvic Rocking is so vital to your comfort and health during pregnancy, here are some additional positions. The hands-and-knees position is by far the most effective means of "rocking your pelvis," so use it whenever possible. These other methods will give variety to your pelvic rocking and can be used during the day as you do your routine activities. You will be able to rock your pelvis when sitting and standing. By maintaining a straight spine with the help of these postures, you will feel infinitely better all day long. No Backache. You are also taking care of the uterus by tipping the pelvis forward from time to time, releasing pressure, and allowing good circulation. These variations count as your daytime pelvic rocking. However, before bed, only the hands-and-knees position is preferred.

You will become dependent on pelvic rocking. At least I have! Nothing makes my back feel so good. I still routinely do my pelvic rocking before bed and have discovered that I maintain a strong back, good posture and tight tummy muscles as a result. I recommend that you, too, consider pelvic rocking a lifetime exercise.

If you are doing these variations in front of others, such as while you sit at your computer at the office, it may look a little less conspicuous if you do them one at a time, with rather long intervals in between. Sitting at your desk, violently working away at pelvic rocking could cause a minor riot at the office. Standing pelvic rocks in front of the filing cabinet will brand you as a belly dancer—at least. These "exercises" are nothing more than basic body movements and can be performed quietly and unobtrusively as a stretch or change of position. They can be used to get attention, though, if you want to teach about Natural Childbirth.

Sitting Pelvic Rock

Though the sitting position is not as effective as the other methods of pelvic rocking, the advantage is that it can be done while you are sitting doing routine tasks. It will relieve back tension and pelvic pressure.

HOW:

1. Begin in a tailor sitting position. Roll your pelvis back so that your weight shifts to the base of your spine. You feel as though you have been pushed in the abdomen.

2. Roll the pelvis forward again as far as it will go. This pushes your abdomen forward.

3. After repeating these motions about ten times, stop when the pelvis is level and relaxed.

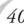

WHERE:

If you are not able to assume a proper tailor sit position on the floor, you can do the pelvic rock sitting in a chair. Not as effective but helps a bit!

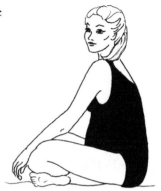

> Try to get yourself out of the habit of crossing your legs when sitting in a chair. This contributes to poor circulation and may also help to build "saddlebags" on the sides of your thighs. An even worse possibility is that it could promote varicose veins or hemorrhoids.

Pelvic rock sitting can be done anywhere: at a desk at the office, at the movies, riding in a car, watching TV, reading, at the computer ... you get the idea. Whenever you are sitting, do occasional pelvic rocks.

WHEN:

Do this mid-morning, noon, mid-afternoon, early evening, and anytime in between. It will be very unobtrusive if done one at a time.

Standing Pelvic Rock

This posture is extremely important since we all stand a great deal, despite our inclinations to the contrary! Standing pelvic rock should be learned so well that your posture will improve. Even if you already have perfect posture you will need to strengthen your muscles to maintain it during a pregnancy. Now is a good time to better your postural habits, since you become uncomfortable so easily carrying your growing baby in your uterus. Standing or sitting or lying with bad posture will give you a backache. So if you have one, use your pelvic rocks. This exercise will not only prevent backaches, it will ease an aching back, also.

+ Standing pelvic rock is especially good for you to build strength in the back muscles so that you can maintain a good posture while standing.

+ It makes you look better because it lifts your chin, raises your breasts, strengthens your shoulders, tightens your buttocks, pulls in your abdomen, and unlocks your knees.

+ You appear to the world as a woman proud to be having a baby.

+ You look and feel two months earlier in pregnancy than you would with a sway-back and a protruding abdomen.

+ You do not outgrow your clothes as quickly; therefore, it is helpful to your clothes budget. You can button your coat and may not have to buy one especially for your pregnancy. (For those of us in cold climates, this is rather important.)

- Standing pelvic rock gives a slight relaxation to the knees and thus aids leg circulation. Varicose vein troubles are decreased.

- Add to all this ... it keeps you from walking like a duck!

- If your back is kept straight it will not ache from the weight of the baby tugging on the muscles and ligaments that connect the uterus to your back.

Some of the stretch of the abdominal wall will be eliminated. One of our class members exemplified how very stretched the abdominal skin can become. She had had three pregnancies prior to taking our classes. Her figure was good, but she had allowed that heavy uterus to pull her abdomen forward. When she did the standing pelvic rock in class for the first time, her dress became tucked between her ribs and abdomen because she had so much stretched loose tissue and skin. She looked so much better and had no back tension after learning this simple posture tip.

The amount of loose skin on your abdomen after the baby is born will depend a great deal on how well you have maintained a good posture throughout your pregnancy. The baby doesn't ruin your figure—you do! If you will use plenty of lubrication on the skin (any kind of skin oil that you like to use) and hold your uterus in your pelvis while standing (keeping buttocks tight), you will have as pretty a figure for a bikini as you ever had ... whether you want to wear one or not.

HOW:

1. Stand facing a chair or any vertical surface. This is only to demonstrate to you how this pelvic rock really makes a difference with your posture.

2. Push your hip and abdomen forward with your tailbone back and up toward the ceiling. Your hand position is not important. Put your hands wherever it is comfortable—shoulders, hips, or down at your side.

3. Now reverse the posture. Tuck your tailbone under you and tighten your buttocks. The top of the pelvis has moved back, bringing the hipbones back, also. Notice how your abdominal wall has tightened and flattened and how much space you now have between your tummy and the chair.

4. Repeat 2 and 3 as many times as you need to make your back feel comfortable.

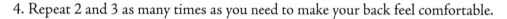

WHERE and WHEN:

Standing pelvic rock can be done anytime you are standing, such as: waiting in line at the supermarket, waiting to cross the street, when you get out of bed (it will help you get moving in the morning!), every time you look in a mirror, when you get out of a car, getting up after sitting on a sofa, and every time you feel tension in your back.

Obviously, this movement can be done any time you wish or remember to do it. It can become such a habit that you'll do it all day long. Eventually your spine will become permanently straight because the muscles are strong and developed. When you are no longer pregnant you should continue to do this to maintain good posture.

"Kitchen Sink" Pelvic Rock or Mabel Fitzhugh's Pelvic Rock

This exercise was taught to me, personally, by Mabel Lumm Fitzhugh, a dear, vivacious, limber lady who was probably in her sixties when I met her. She spent several days with us when I was being trained as a new teacher. Dr. Bradley had her come to Denver to help us reevaluate our program. This exercise was added to our pelvic rock variations at that time. Its special quality is that it can be easily fitted into a busy day.

The "Kitchen Sink" can be anything of the right height—a chair back at the office, the desktop in the schoolroom, a window ledge, bathroom sink, countertop, cupboard, dresser, etc.—wherever you are. We suggest the kitchen sink because it is a spot where you will spend much time if you are a homemaker. The exercise should be done each time you go to the sink (or to the chair at your desk, etc.). Through frequent practice you will maintain good posture, give yourself quick relief from pelvic pressure, and you will improve circulation to the lower part of your body.

Mrs. Fitzhugh used this exercise as a test on pregnant women in a clinic where no other form of exercise was encouraged. The women showed a marked avoidance of varicose veins and much less back discomfort than a control group.

HOW:

1. Stand straight about two feet away from the sink, with feet comfortably apart (about six inches). Distances will depend upon your size.

2. Bow to the sink! In other words, bend from the hips with a straight back.

3. Put your hands on the edge of the counter, elbows stiff, and let your hands support your weight. That is, lean into your hands.

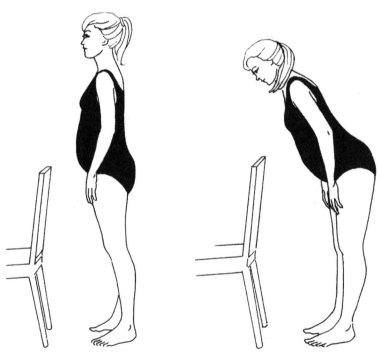

4. Point your tailbone toward the ceiling. It may hurt behind your knees, so go easy!

5. Tuck your tailbone down and under you, as you relax your knees. This rolls your hipbones backward as your spine gets a comfortable stretch.

6. Do Step 4 and Step 5, three times very slowly.

7. Now, with your lower back rounded, your tailbone tucked under you, knees relaxed, and buttocks tight, straighten your shoulders and head over the rest of your body. Be sure to keep the good posture that you have created in the lower part of your back.

8. Walk up to the counter and find that you can get four inches closer to it! Keep your knees relaxed and the same pelvic posture as you go on to do other things.

9. Repeat each time you go to the sink! Decide what you will use as your "kitchen sink" that will be your reminder to do this often during your busy day.

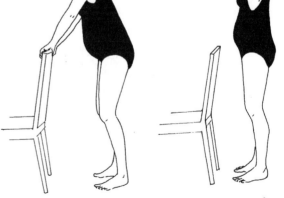

WHERE:

This can be done at any table, counter, or desk that is the right height for you. If the counter is about the height of the top of your pelvic bone—about two inches below your waist—it is just right.

WHEN:

Do this exercise all day long, every time you go to your kitchen sink—or whatever chair or ledge you decide on as your point of most frequency during the day.

Rhondda's Tip

Knowing about and integrating pelvic rocks in your daily routine will change your physical and mental life. Make pelvic rocks part of your regular routine, just like brushing your teeth. Why? Simply this: doing pelvic rocks during and long after your pregnancy ends will enhance your life. Your back muscles will be stronger … your body will be the better for it.

Chapter 4

Relaxation ... Get Ready for Loose and Limp!

The meaning of the word "relaxation" as we will use it in Natural Childbirth may be very different from your past experience. It is a skill that you will find useful for the rest of your life. Here is what the word means to me and to you too from now on.

Relaxation takes mental activity to keep you physically inactive. In other words, you work hard with your mind to keep your body still and quiet! It is very different from actual sleep, when our minds probably fall asleep before our bodies relax. Relaxing takes mental discipline, especially while the uterus is in hard contraction. During relaxation as used in labor, there is absolutely no sleepiness involved but rather a much heightened awareness and complete control over oneself. You may even think of yourself as "working hard" at relaxing. Remember, it is very passive work physically but hard work mentally.

Relaxation must be considered the most important factor in an enjoyable childbirth experience. *Relaxing is the crux of Natural Childbirth.* The only help you can give the uterus with its work in the first stage of labor is to relax ... let it be. Get out of the way! Do not interfere. To do this requires tremendous concentration because the uterus contracts to a hard knot with each contraction. It is a sensation that you can ease your body through if you're relaxed, but what a difference if you are tense! The uterine contraction has many times greater intensity when the muscles surrounding it are also tense and tight.

I've done it five times in childbirth and know that it is so—but you may be skeptical. Each one of you may try it for yourself. It is a very easy theory to prove in labor. Just tighten any group of muscles while you are in the middle of a contraction. For example, make a fist with one hand. You will be convinced that you are having amuch harder contraction than you were having previously. It works every time. Try this small experiment whileyou are in early labor so it will not hurt too much.

The theory of why relaxation makes your contractions feel better is explained in *Husband-Coached Childbirth* published by Robert Bradley.

Dr. Bradley said:

Now we come to a facet of humans that is inescapable. There is a relationship between mind and body which is the psychosomatic nature of humans. The mind and body are interacting, one helping or hindering the other. It is probably impossible to relax the body completely if the mind is under tension. Vice versa, it is impossible to relax the mind completely if the body is under tension. This is observed also in animals in their need to concentrate during labor and the temporary viciousness of laboring animals if this concentration is disrupted in any way.

My second labor began at a La Leche League meeting at the home of Mary Ann Kerwin, one of the co-founders of La Leche League. I called Richard to come for me so we could go on to the hospital from there. Things were going well. I was relaxed on a sofa, feeling as though we had lots of time, so Richard and Tom Kerwin had some cake and coffee, left from the meeting refreshments.

There was much conversation and laughter, the four of us being rather excited. It was a joke in the middle of a contraction that changed my attitude. When I tried to laugh, I realized that my contractions were very strong is and hard and we'd better not dawdle too long. Relaxing too well can fool you! I did have enough time for my daughter Claryss Nan to make her official debut in the hospital with the doctor in attendance as planned.

The point of this incident is that you may feel so comfortable you'll not know that your relaxing is responsible for your comfort and that your labor is actually hard. Laughing, coughing, or trying to be polite and answer a nurse—any activity in the middle of a contraction will prove to you by contrast that relaxation works. You will also find out that not doing it right for one contraction does not ruin your whole labor. Just get back into your good relaxing technique and you will have a wonderful experience in your first stage of labor. In second stage of labor we do something quite different.

Just remember that any part of your body in tension is going to add tension to the uterine contraction. That means it will hurt! That is why most people call a contraction a "labor pain." It also detracts from the efficiency of the contracting uterus. That means your labor could be longer. Stay out of the way and let the uterus do its work. You'll feel better and the labor will not be slowed down.

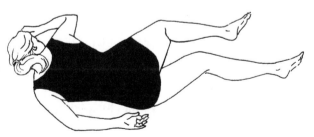

HOW:

Classic Position—Lie on your side on a firm padded surface with one arm under and behind you, the other bent in front of your face. Both legs are bent at the knee, the upper one pulled forward to help support the weight of your body away from the baby.

51

Pillows may be used wherever necessary to make you more comfortable—under your knee, under your leg and foot or under your head and chest to help hold your weight off the lower shoulder, or both by using two pillows. Make yourself comfortable. Every part of your body should be supported. Try putting a pillow under your head then pull the corner of the pillow down between your breasts. If that does not feel good then keep adjusting until it works for you. Relaxation is impossible if you are not in a comfortable position as you begin.

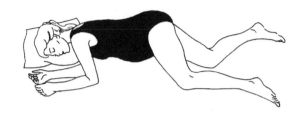

Variation of Classic Position—Your arms may be more comfortable in front, but avoid putting one arm on top of the other or holding your head on your arms, which creates a point of tension.

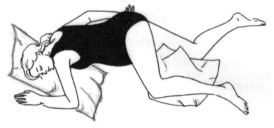

Contour Position—Each part of the body is supported with pillows to prevent tension. This position may be useful during transition. I used it exclusively during transition. Please make sure that you are not lying flat on your back. You must elevate upper body to a forty-five degree angle. There must not be pressure on the blood vessels within the pelvis which would compromise blood flow to the uterus.

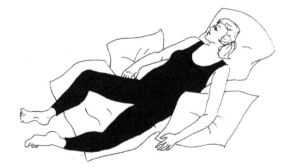

To prepare for relaxation, especially during labor, keep in mind these necessary conditions:

1. The proper atmosphere includes absence of strangers, solitude, and a quiet, restful room with as little unexpected noise or commotion as possible. Avoid a glaring light, but a soft, dull light will probably be comfortable. Set the stage for this event. Make the environment suit you. It will enhance your relaxation and make your birth an amazingly wonderful experience.

2. Use the comfortable positions, as shown. These basic positions vary some with each individual. Just make sure that each joint is slightly bent, not straight or fully flexed. Position your body and use pillows to help you become comfortable with all tension relieved. If you are in labor in a hospital, the bed will adjust to help with your positioning. Do not let any one part of the body bear the weight of any other part of the body. In other words, don't have your head resting on your arm, or one leg on the other.

3. Control your breathing. Use slow, steady, and relaxed abdominal breathing. I will discuss this technique fully later on.

4. Complete concentration and attention to what you are doing is imperative. Closing your eyes helps you control your environment. You shut it out and ignore everything!

Get Ready for Loose and Limp!

Now, assume the classic position and get yourself as comfortable and relaxed as you can. If you then have your husband/coach read the poem I've written, you should be able to relax even more. You'll soon observe how you respond to different words and phrases and begin to think creatively about what other words or routines might be better for you. If you wish to begin at the toes and work up the body that is as good as using the baby as the focal point the way I have done. You may prefer to use a "total body" idea of relaxing and not go to the progressive method at all. Perhaps you will do best with "pleasant thought" or meditative relaxing.

My husband, with his gift of words, was marvelous at relaxing me. I did not have to teach him how. He knew how to relax himself. You will benefit in labor if you teach your husband to relax now. Try it out with him. Prove to him how relaxing it is to speak softly and lovingly. Show him how hard it is to keep tension in his face when you are offering suggestions of a relaxed face. Demonstrate how a bad position hinders his relaxing. Test out words and touching to see how he responds. When he has learned to relax, he will be better able to coach you to perfect relaxation. It is also a good idea for you to see how hard it is to be in the coaching role. You will be a much better team after this reversal of roles.

One couple had spent time together working and planning for the labor. He had given careful thought to helping his wife relax and when the time came for the real thing, they did very well. During one of the contractions, the father-to-be became either tired or excited, probably both, and as part of the relaxing monologue said, "Now, relax your hair." That was the end of relaxation with that contraction, as she burst into giggles. He used more sensible suggestions for relaxing during the remainder of their labor.

I offer what I have used effectively for years as a way of easily teaching others to relax—often a very new skill for many people in our fast-living society. So, begin with this and then progress to your own variation. Even if you continue to use my words, you will place your own meaning on them. Relaxing is so personal that I can only teach it the way I feel it. Try to tune in with me and let it work for you.

Have your husband or your coach read or "croon" this to you slowly and quietly as a poem or a lullaby, giving time for it to take effect:

Loose and Limp ... Warm and Heavy

Let your whole being
Sink slowly, slowly, slowly.
Feel your muscles
Become limp and loose and comfortable.
Drifting or floating,
Relaxed and comfortable,
warmth and heaviness spread through your body.
The baby in your uterus
is warm and heavy.
Feel warmth and heaviness
spreading from the baby to your abdomen, hips,
thighs, knees, lower legs, ankles,
feet and toes.
Slowly, quietly
the lower half of you is
loose and limp, warm and heavy.
The upper half of you awaits its turn.
Slowly release, let go, warm and heavy,
limp and loose.

Let every cell absorb and enjoy,
spreading up your back and front,
chest and shoulders.
Arms and fingers let go.

As your neck releases tension,
your head slowly shifts and becomes
more and more relaxed.
Nearer and nearer that comfortable state of
relaxation.

Erase the worries from your brow,
eyes loose but closed.
Eyes and all around eyes
limp and loose.
Cheeks loosen and droop,
jaw drops.
Tongue is loose in your mouth,
lips part slightly.
Warm, heavy, and comfortable.
Deep, slow, heavy breathing.
Breathe in and out slowly,

abdomen up and down slowly.
Limp and loose,
warm and heavy,
comfortably relaxed.

In your mind's eye
hold a softly purring kitten in your lap
while sunshine warms you both.
Listen to the laughter of children
sledding on a crisp sparkly snowy hill.
Ride a bicycle on a lazy autumn afternoon,
hair blowing in the wind.
Sit before a roaring, snapping fire
a crisp apple ready to eat.
Watch a robin build her nest,
weaving string and straw with precision.
Lie on the warm sand, you and your love,
while the waves roll up on the beach.

Limp and loose,
warm and heavy,
comfortably relaxed.

WHERE and WHEN:

You will relax completely and breathe abdominally during each contraction in the first stage of labor. In between contractions you will not need to relax. Preparing for labor will take much practice, so relax whenever you can lie down for a nap and every night as you go to bed. It takes only minutes and will help you relax for sleep.

One good way to test yourself is to spend two minutes on the floor with a soft rug at the busiest time of your day. You may have a toddler pulling at your eyelids and asking, "Are you asleep, Mommy?" That is very good preparation for labor, when you must ignore your environment and concentrate on yourself. As I was getting ready to go to the hospital in my third labor, our two-year-old, Claryss Nan, did just that! She tried to open myeyes as I relaxed.

So I mean what I say! Explain to your wee ones what you are doing and why. Have them relax with you if they will. Set your timer for two minutes and relax. Put up with the crawling over you, the riding on your back and the noisy toddlers in the next room, whatever. Labor may even seem easy by comparison! If you have a tendency to fall asleep and sleep for hours, despite what is going on around you, do set your alarm!

Warning:
Falling asleep is not good relaxing practice. You have stopped concentrating on your relaxation or you'd never fall asleep. So stay awake and think hard about relaxing.

You can relax at other times, too, of course. I do think it best to lie down, but sometimes you could sit in a chair and try to loosen your body as much as possible. Any efforts to relax will help you become better at it.

Although you are learning to relax so that your labor will be easier, this may be the most important technique you will learn for improving your quality of life. Tension and sleeplessness are big problems in our modern society. You have it solved by knowing how to relax intentionally.

It works spectacularly with children. Are your children rowdy at bedtime? Just use your relaxing voice and words to calm them down. It's magic!

When I am teaching Relaxing Techniques at the Bradley Method Teachers Training, there are multiple little ones crawling around. Of course they hate it when their mother lies down, closes her eyes and begins to relax. The child feels ignored. For a few minutes there is mild confusion. I begin my soft, crooning relaxing words. The mother will usually put a comforting hand on the child and soon everyone becomes comfortable and quiet. Moms and babies calmly relax. It always works!

Sometimes when you are very good at relaxing you will feel as though you have fallen asleep but it is really an altered state of consciousness. It is sometimes called *blissed out*. It's a lovely experience and I hope you have it happen to you. However it is not likely to happen during labor. You will need to work very hard to keep your body loose and limp all the while your uterus is contracting extremely hard. During labor, your contractions will rarely last more than a minute. In between them you can change position or stretch. In very hard labor, you may even fall asleep in between contractions and when the next one wakes you, concentrate on your relaxing and go back to serious abdominal breathing.

Think of relaxation as a form of meditation.

Rhondda's Tip

Practicing for two minutes is good preparation to do well with actual labor contractions. If you are not relaxing with abdominal breathing, you could feel as though you have continuous contractions in the transition of labor. Believe me, your body could not actually do that. Contractions come and go. Work with your body and you will get good at this before you actually need it in labor.

Chapter 5

The Secret of Abdominal Breathing

During the first stage of labor, with each contraction you will breathe with your abdomen and relax completely. Between contractions you may do what you feel like doing and breathe comfortably. Abdominal breathing and relaxation belong together. You do them better together than you are able to do each separately. Your ability to do both will increase with practice, so the amount of time you spend at it beforehand will pay great dividends during labor.

I have already discussed relaxation and referred to abdominal breathing. Now we will learn the basics of abdominal breathing and from then on you should do the two together.

When you breathe abdominally, you have the feeling that great amounts of air are being pulled into your abdominal cavity. This is impossible, of course. What is happening is that the diaphragm is pulling down into the abdomen so that the lungs can expand fully. The diaphragm is a muscle which acts as a bellow. It pulls down and air is sucked into the lungs. It pushes up and the lungs are emptied. Naturally, the bigger the amounts of air you take into your lungs, the slower your breathing will be and the higher your abdominal wall will rise.

When you inhale, your abdomen rises—as you exhale, it lowers. The breathing must be very slow and full. Give plenty of time for each part of the breath.

Since your body will be working very hard during labor, you will require great quantities of oxygen to fulfill your needs. At the same time, you must be totally relaxed for your labor to progress smoothly and easily. I do not recommend that you do this, but if you ran around the outside of your house, then put yourself into a relaxation position and practiced abdominal breathing, you would get the feeling of the kind of breathing required during labor. You would also notice that you needed your mouth open to get enough breath. Your muscles must be relaxed but your body is working hard and therefore requires big deep breaths. So when we say, "Relax and breathe slowly and deeply," the effect in practice will be different from the real thing in labor.

Raising the abdominal wall as high as possible is important in labor for another reason. The uterus, as it tightens with a contraction, will bulge. This pushes it against the abdominal wall. Now, if your abdominal muscles are relaxed and being raised slowly with abdominal breathing, there will be minimal discomfort when the contracting, bulging uterus pushes against the abdominal wall. Pull tight on the abdominal muscles and see the tension created between two hard, contracted muscles—the uterus and the abdomen. Make sure you remember this when you are in labor.

Relaxing with abdominal breathing keeps the abdominal muscles soft and relaxed and slowly pushed away from the contracting uterus by your big oxygen-laden inhalation. During exhalation, the abdominal wall along with the whole body remains relaxed to avoid interference with the work of the contracting uterus.

It is so simple and makes such good sense! You are trying to let the uterus do its work by staying out of its way. At the same time you must supply it with necessary materials. Deep breathing will supply the necessary amounts of oxygen to the blood. A good position allows adequate circulation to the uterus so the blood supply reaches it. The side-lying position best serves this need. However, the contour position is a possible variation. Remember that lots of stretching and moving about between contractions will help keep you comfortable.

Abdominal breathing is necessary

First … you need the large amount of oxygen that this type of deep breathing will allow. Ordinary breathing, usually much more shallow, cannot easily serve the great oxygen needs of the laboring body.

Secondly … you can relax much better if you breathe in this manner, and only with relaxation will you be comfortable during first-stage labor.

Thirdly … the control used in the breathing helps give you the mastery of your body required to "ride" with each contraction of the uterus. You are the director of this show!

HOW:

1. Recline in a contour position with knees raised to lessen the tension of the abdominal muscles. This position is for learning how, more than for labor. As soon as you have learned the technique, you may practice on your side in a relaxed position.

2. Put hands low on abdomen so that you can feel the pubic bone. This guides you to take a deeper breath than if your hands are higher up on the abdomen.

3. Open your mouth and take a deep breath. Let the breath push your abdomen and hands up.

4. Slowly let your breath out and hands and abdomen go down again.

5. Repeat and practice for about two minutes. Breathe slowly and deeply.

6. Now put one hand up on your chest. There should be no chest movement as you continue to breathe abdominally.

Stop and rest! Now do it again, and make each breath as long in duration as is comfortable. Try to "fill your abdomen" with air. Notice the difference between letting the breath push your abdomen up and having the muscles lift your abdomen.

You *must not* tense your muscles. For you to be comfortable in labor, your abdominal wall must remain relaxed while the uterus is contracting. Sometimes this can be a confusing thing but your husband will be able to feel the difference with his hand and can coach you to know when you are doing well. Practice together now so that you'll be a good team when labor begins. He could read Dr. Bradley's *Husband-Coached Childbirth* to aid him in his understanding of the coach's role.

WHERE:

Where do you practice? In bed, as you lie down for an afternoon rest (it is a lovely idea, isn't it?) and when you are ready for sleep at night. Do several minutes of concentrated relaxation with abdominal breathing each time.

Begin to use abdominal breathing during the day as you think of it. As you first learn this type of breathing, you may despair that it will ever become easy. It quickly becomes a comfortable way of breathing, though, and by the time you go into labor, it should come very naturally. The more you practice, the easier your first stage of labor will be. When your labor reaches an intensity that demands your attention start relaxing and abdominal breathing with each contraction until the first stage of labor is completed and you are ready to begin pushing.

WHEN:

During pregnancy—Practice often during pregnancy, at least three times each day, taking several breaths. Consider two minutes a good amount of time for a practice contraction, although a contraction would not likely be this long—one minute to one and one-half minutes is more likely, even at transition (end of the first stage).

You will soon learn to breathe abdominally in other positions so that you can practice it all day long. Practice it while sitting in a contour position until you know for sure how to do it, and then alternate with the side-lying relaxation position.

In labor—With each contraction, relax completely and take deep, slow, full abdominal breaths. Continue with abdominal breathing and relaxation for the total time of each contraction. In between you can stretch, move, talk or even go to sleep. With the next contraction, go back to "work" immediately.

Rhondda's Tip

Any time you have the opportunity to lie down, practice abdominal breathing. As your pregnancy advances and your uterus and belly expand, knowing how to maximize your breathing will not only benefit you overall, it will ease your labor.

Chapter 6

Squatting Gets the Job Done

Let's face it squatting is not a ladylike posture, think of it as "mother-like." It is important, so use it proudly. The squat is the position you will assume to give birth. It opens the "baby door," the pelvis is pulled as wide open as it can get. So get busy and limber up those squatting muscles! Many a mother, alas, has been instructed or forced to "hold her legs together" until the doctor or midwife arrived, to keep her baby from being born. This is effective in preventing birth—painfully. Therefore, the opposite holds true for hastening birth. The wider apart you hold your legs, the sooner the baby can be born—joyfully.

Squatting is healthy because it permits light and air to this region of your body. It is helpful in preventing yeast infections. To induce the growth of yeast, four key conditions are required: damp, dark, moist and reduced oxygen. When your legs are held together, you create the perfect medium.

It also develops better circulation in the perineal area, which leads to better muscle tone and healthier tissue. By squatting, you are preparing the perineum to stretch better to allow the birth of your baby.

If an episiotomy becomes necessary—cutting of the perineum during crowning to facilitate the baby's passage— healing will be much faster and easier because you have been squatting throughout your pregnancy.

HOW:

Bend your knees as you lower into a squat position, keep your heels on the floor and your toes straight ahead. Keep weight on the outer edges of your feet as much as possible. Place your arms between your knees so that your shoulders and knees are close together.

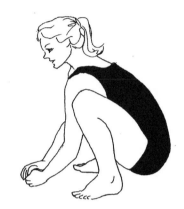

Use this position only as long as it is comfortable—actually, very short times. Even if you can stay in the squat position for a longer time, be careful, as you may feel "fused" into a squat position before you know it.

If you cannot balance and you keep falling back into a sitting position, hold on to a heavy object such as the bottom of a chest of drawers, a bed leg, the lower cupboards in the kitchen, the bottom of a closed door—anything that will support you and yet keep your hands low enough to maintain a proper squat position. It will help you if your clothes are loose or stretchy. You might find it easier to balance while you are learning to squat, if you wear shoes. The bit of a lift from the heel of the shoes will help you balance.

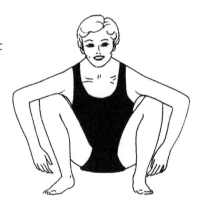

There is another way to learn to squat by pairing with someone else. Each of you acts as a counter-weight to the other. Grasp your partner's wrists; then slowly lower yourselves while at the same time pulling against the body weight of your partner. Your back remains straight and your arms are outstretched. Keep lowering yourselves to the squat position. Maintain it by leaning your shoulders forward between your knees.

If squatting is difficult for you, do not be discouraged. Keep trying, using all these helpful tricks and you will be squatting with ease in no time!

Getting up from a squat—
HOW:

To come up to a standing position, push your tailbone toward the ceiling as your legs straighten, then raise the upper portion of your body upright. Use your hands on your thighs to help push yourself up. This helps tilt the heavy uterus up and out of the pelvis. It is a variation of the pelvic rock—think of it as a vertical pelvic rock.

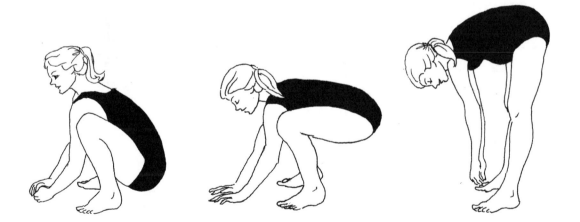
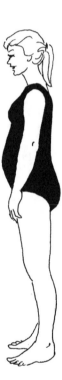

Lifting from a Squat to protect your back—

Warning: you must *not* lift any weight from a squat position as you come up from the floor using your back, as we do in the normal squat. It is a nice pelvic rock to add but you are using your back for this maneuver.

Therefore, when lifting anything heavier than an article of clothing from the floor, use your legs … not your back. Your back has enough of a load with your pregnant tummy to lift.

HOW:

After you are in the squat position, change your posture from the squat to the position with your feet diagonal that is one in front of the other which creates a much larger base and gives you better balance.

During pregnancy, women need a broader base to balance their extra weight.

It's not an equal distribution and it's concentrated primarily around the expanding uterus.

Notice the area of floor if you draw an imaginary square around your feet; compare this area with that of an ordinary squat. Keep your back straight as you use your leg muscles to lift yourself into a standing posture. Since pregnancy sometimes causes slight dizziness as you change position, a chair or table

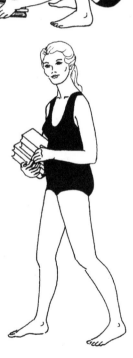

nearby can be grasped with one hand to steady you. If you are lifting a heavy object remember to use your legs, not your back. As a mother you will be lifting often!

This is also a useful posture for reaching the baby in a crib or bassinet. Use your legs and keep your back straight. No reason to cause extra back strain and discomfort.

WHERE and WHEN:

Squat anytime you find it necessary to reach low: getting into lower cupboards, gardening, picking up laundry or light objects, caring for children, changing diapers, tying shoes, loving, hugging, or talking to a child, helping dress, buttoning, showing things, explaining, etc.

You may have to restrict this position to times and places when you are alone—or risk being laughed at. I vividly recall using this posture as a matter of habit when I was ten years old, until my friends embarrassed me by laughing at my lack of sophistication. When I was in college, however, it became fashionable to squat— we called it "hunkering." You may or may not be acceptable to others around you when you use this posture, so you must have conviction about how good it is for you.

Rhondda's Tip

The squat is a lifetime habit for you to learn. When not pregnant, you can rise from the original squat position with your back straight, since you do not have a heavy uterus to overbalance you. It is much easier and more graceful.

Chapter 7

The Glory of Kegel!

Kegel Exercise—Tightening the Pubococcygeus Muscle

There isn't a muscle in your body identified as a Kegel—it's named after a gynecologist who discovered that an easy series of "squeezes" within the lower pelvic area of a woman's body had incredible benefits.

The pubococcygeus muscle is the floor of the pelvis, encompassing the perineal area. As its name indicates, it includes the area from the pubis, in front, to the coccyx, or tailbone, in back. It is the muscle that allows you to control the three openings all women have: the opening from the bladder (urethra), the opening from the uterus (vagina), and the opening from the bowel (rectum).

Try to open or tighten each of these separately and you will find it impossible. They all work together because this one muscle controls the whole area. Your goal is to learn to be conscious of the control of the pubococcygeus muscle, and especially to maintain a constant tension in it. You will call this "Kegeling."

All the organs in the abdomen rest on this layer of muscle. You can imagine how incredibly important that makes it! If it is weak, everything shifts. You could have loss of bladder and bowel control, also your sex life and birth experience would suffer.

Instead of the pubococcygeus muscle, most women know of it as the "Kegel muscle" and exercising that muscle is the "Kegel exercise," named after Dr. Arnold Kegel, the former director of the Kegel Clinic at

Los Angeles County, USC Medical Clinic, who worked until his death to help women understand their own functions.

I had the opportunity to hear this handsome, white-haired, soft-spoken gentleman tell how he had begun his work in 1950s by trying to prevent prolapse of the uterus in his gynecology patients. He taught them to squeeze the muscle that contracted the vaginal walls in an attempt to strengthen the support for the uterus.

His patients responded as he'd hoped. After several months of exercising, they showed stronger muscular support in the perineum, which prevented further prolapse or *falling* of the uterus. His patients began to disclose further benefits. There was a bonus … rather surreptitiously, they admitted that their sex life had improved. Dr. Kegel began to document the functions of the pubococcygeus muscle and started his lifelong crusade to help females understand how their bodies function and how to prevent physical inadequacy with a simple exercise.

> The role of Kegel exercise and muscle is vital during pregnancy, postpartum and for the rest of your life.

Kegeling during Pregnancy, Birth and After Delivery

Most women have learned about the Kegel exercise at some time—few realize how it will affect their lives. Here is how important it is:

+ *During pregnancy*, the extra weight of the uterus stretches the pubococcygeus, which makes exercising it for strength very important. You know that a muscle which is used constantly is able to stretch and return to normal without injury and also is much stronger. A good healthy muscle, having good tone, will be able to support a growing uterus for nine months and return to its usual function and strength after the birth.

+ *During the birth process*, the Kegel muscle is put to a great test. It must have enough elasticity to move high into the vaginal wall and not impede the descent of the baby. When you relax this muscle while pushing, you do not slow the birth. If you tighten it during a pushing contraction it will cause discomfort and pain and could slow the progress of labor.

+ *After delivery*, the flexing of the Kegel muscle helps healing in general, and episiotomy healing in particular, if an episiotomy was performed. Healing is supported by the increase of blood supply to this area of your body. The same would be true for a tear in the perineum.

+ *For the Rest of Your Life*, contracting and relaxing this muscle brings improved circulation to all the tissues in the area. It keeps the muscle healthy and strong to support the abdominal contents. All of the reasons for using this exercise during pregnancy are valid for the rest of your life. See below!

Stress incontinence during pregnancy is not uncommon—i.e., you may have a slight leakage of urine when you cough, sneeze or jump. This problem is effectively cured with "Kegeling."

For the rest of your life, the good condition of this muscle needs to be maintained. The proper alignment of your pelvic and abdominal organs depends ultimately on the Kegel muscle. An improper position, or a sagging or falling of the uterus, is called *prolapsed uterus, fallen womb,* or sometimes *tipped uterus.*

There are many names but it all begins with a uterus that is not exactly where it belongs. The symptoms are backache, heaviness in the pelvis, bladder infections, frequency of urination, incontinence, cystocele and rectocele. These are all problems of aging so keep Kegeling throughout your life.

What is cystocele and rectocele? Here's a simplified explanation. As the uterus pushes downward into the pelvis, it pulls the adjacent tissues with it. This causes the tubes from the bladder (urethra) and the bowel (rectum) to get into abnormal positions. Pockets can form which make complete emptying of the bladder and bowel difficult. There is increased risk of infections as urine becomes "caught" in a pocket or cystocele. A pocket in the rectum (rectocele) causes alternate constipation (which may help develop hemorrhoids) and diarrhea as the blockage finally releases.

I have purposely listed these unpleasant "women's complaints" because the good tone of your Kegel muscle can prevent them. Kegel to keep everything up and in where it belongs.

Now, need I remind you about your bonus? Your sexual satisfaction is another good measure of how well you've done your Kegels! By the way, this is a good exercise for men, too.

I had been teaching this exercise and using Dr. Kegel's name for years before I finally had the opportunity to hear him speak. I was very impressed by his soft humor and completely "proper" attitude to a subject that just begged for off-color remarks. As he was explaining a point, he put his hand into his jacket pocket and pulled out a small white box. Opening it, he removed some cotton packing—as would be used with jewelry—and very gently pulled out the cast of a female vagina. I was speechless!

He had developed a plastic which he could pour into a vagina that would harden and set instantly and could be removed easily. He then had an exact model and could show the "owner" her problems. If the pubococcygeus muscle was in good tone, with proper tension maintained, the vagina resembled a cylinder. If the lady's muscle was a mess, her vagina was more like a thick pancake.

Think about it … would your partner want a smooth cylinder or a flat tire when your sex life resumed after childbirth? What a teacher he was! How could a lesson like that ever be forgotten? It still makes me laugh.

HOW:

Tighten the "stopping the flow of urine" muscle. Now, as you tighten, pull up or lift with the tightening. "Tighten—lift—lift—hold—let—go."

Count it so that with each tightening you lift to the count of three, hold for one count and relax to the count of two. The whole count takes about two seconds. This will help teach you the constant tension that should be present in this muscle. It should never be completely relaxed while you are awake.

The first times you try this, spread your legs slightly apart, then tighten and release the muscle. Do not allow other muscles to get involved. Buttocks, thighs, and abdomen can be confused at first with the simple Kegel contraction.

Since the Kegel muscle can control the flow of urine, try to interrupt the flow when you are voiding. Use this only as test to see how well you are tightening your muscle. Since the baby is now bouncing about on your bladder you will need a strong Kegel. You will notice that you do not need to empty your bladder as often with a stronger muscle. Your bathroom visits during the night might decrease, too.

WHERE:

Anywhere—any position. No one should be able to see you using this muscle as long as you are doing it correctly—unless you are like one gal in class who claimed that she could not do the Kegel without opening and closing her mouth, fishlike, at the same time. There really is no physical connection.

Hear "Kegel"... squeeze and lift!

Talking on the phone is a good time to do twenty. You can brush your teeth and Kegel, watch TV and Kegel, stand in the supermarket line and Kegel, wait for a stoplight and Kegel, hold the door open for children and Kegel, read your emails and Kegel, pelvic rock and Kegel, stir the soup and Kegel, read this and Kegel!!

WHEN:

Twenty times each waking hour for the rest of your life. In other words, only when you are asleep should your Kegel muscle relax.

To remind yourself to do your Kegels someone devised a system of colored sticky dots or notes put here and there around the house. Every time you pass it, you do some Kegels. You could have them on the cupboard door, a mirror, the top of the stairs, on a hallway wall, on your steering wheel, your purse … you get the idea. They will not have to be labeled. You will know what they mean!

How Can Your Coach Help?

Use your imagination and good humor and I'm sure that together, you'll find a variety of pleasant ways to exercise the mighty Kegel.

Rhondda's Tip

To Kegel or not to Kegel … that should **never** be the question!

Chapter 8

The *Natural* of Natural Childbirth Is Up to You

By the end of the third month, you've worked through most of those early new feelings about being pregnant. You are becoming comfortable with your new state of being. It's still exciting, but not so scary. Your tummy is still a bit small for many of the fashionable maternity clothes available to you. However, you know—you cannot wear everything in your closet anymore. If this is not your first pregnancy, you will "show" sooner and become bigger than you did with your first pregnancy.

You've noticed other changes in your body. Your breasts may be tender and enlarging. You may have darkened pigment on your face and nipples as well as a line down the center of your lovely barely bulging tummy.

Most of you will have finished with that awful nausea, but if not, you've discovered that it is not going to get any better by thinking you are sick, so you are trying to ignore it. Few offer any sympathy for it anymore either. Your spouse or partner is probably as tired of it as you are. Because this is an issue for some of you, I'll offer you some tips on how to deal with this in a later chapter, *Problems of Pregnancy ... Heartburn and Nausea.*

Your baby is kicking now. It is exciting to know that those movements in your abdomen that you thought were intestinal grumblings are probably the baby bumping around. He is still terribly small—about seven inches and four ounces—but he is a complete being. That's a lot of development in four months.

The baby's birth seems so far off, yet you feel as though you've been pregnant forever! It's a good time to work harder practicing your relaxation and abdominal breathing.

Getting Started with Natural Childbirth

You've been getting many questions about Natural Childbirth from all directions. You are now really aware of how necessary it is to be able to explain what you are planning to do. Your husband or partner, too, may be getting lots of comment, which may have either turned him into a fanatic or made him a little suspicious. The two of you may need to study up a bit on the subject.

One of the classics is the book written by Dr. Robert Bradley. In *Husband-Coached Childbirth,* he reveals his philosophy behind Natural Childbirth and a variety of methods of effective coaching throughout pregnancy and during childbirth itself.

Check my website, *NaturalChildbirthExercises.com* for classic and current readings that will be instructive and helpful. I will be updating and adding to the resources listed on my website as they come to my attention. The classics will be there and will not change. The more you know and understand about pregnancy and birth, the better.

Remember that Natural Childbirth is Educated Childbirth!
Find a Bradley Method Class and join it!
READ, READ, READ.

Find a Bradley Method Class and Join!

Have you researched the Bradley Method online to find an affiliated teacher near you? That is your first step in the education for Natural Childbirth … after reading this book!

Pregnancy is an exclusive club—almost like a secret society. There is a pleasant, friendly feeling among you and other pregnant women. You recognize a common bond with each other—that secret handshake. This is an excellent time to be in a class with other parents who are excited about Natural Childbirth. You know by now that the whole world is not appreciative of Natural Childbirth. You are probably trying to talk everyone you know into having a baby "our right" way and it is fun to find that others in the class are doing the same.

As a matter of fact, almost everything one of you says has the rest of the group nodding their heads in agreement. It is very validating to be in a group as you progress in pregnancy. I am sorry if classes are not possible for you for any reason. If that is the case for you, as a mom-to-be, you must find a chat room or blog on the internet that deals with pregnancy, birth and babies. Connect with others … others just like you with the same aches and pains and hopes and dreams and questions … lots of them.

I highly recommend that you find a supportive health care provider who will support and encourage you as you use *Natural Childbirth Exercises* as your guide. The value of the exercises has been tested for decades. It is critical that you believe in the rights and responsibilities that you have as parents of this tiny child about to be born into your family. The wrong information will be unhelpful—choose your classes and reading carefully.

Choose your health care provider with great care. Do not be a wimp. Find the best one for you and one that believes as you do about the birth. Liking the person is not enough! You need a strong decision maker with power who will advocate for you when you are in the middle of labor being bullied by the nurses to do what you did not want in your birth experience! It will be too late to fire your doctor when as you are in hard labor! Make the decision early and choose wisely. Remember, you are doing the hiring and paying for it, too.

Rhondda's Tip

You are your own best advocate; you must become an expert on Natural Childbirth! Take responsibility for this very important event in your life.

Chapter 9

Problems of Pregnancy ... Heartburn and Nausea

Yes, Virginia, there are some problems of pregnancy! Let's discuss a few.

Heartburn

For many of you, heartburn will be a problem of pregnancy. It is generally avoided by proper diet and yet there are times when your healthy dinner and your baby seem to be fighting for space—which is exactly what is happening. Heartburn is just what it says: a burning sensation at the level of the heart. It is indigestion which you may feel from your stomach all the way up to your throat along the esophagus and it can be very uncomfortable. Unfortunately, it may come and go throughout the second half of your pregnancy.

The hormones produced by the placenta cause the smooth muscles to relax all along the digestive system and this includes the valve into the stomach. The relaxed valve allows acid from the stomach to seep and splash up into the esophagus causing the burning sensation. These same hormones slow the movement of food through your system during pregnancy. Some changes in your eating will be necessary to keep you comfortable!

The first way to try to get rid of heartburn is to get up and move around. Since it usually happens when you lie down, this is in itself an irritation. If you are sitting in a chair or lying down watching television, for example, it is sure to get worse. If you are still bothered after moving around, then try this:

1. Put your hands on your ribs at your sides.

2. Open your mouth and take deep, heavy breaths, pushing your ribs against your hands as they rest on your side.

3. Do this several times, at least 10.

In this way, you give your stomach a bit more space, allowing proper digestion to begin.

Do I need to tell you to eat small, frequent meals? A daily portion of yogurt (about one-quarter cup) seems to help prevent heartburn in many cases. Sometimes a mint or chewing gum is helpful. Often a few sips of milk will bring comfort.

Pregnancy is not a great time to embrace the use of antacids. Avoid them—antacids aren't your friends. The old fashioned cure for heart burn was bicarbonate of soda. That same soda will neutralize the acid which is splashing into your esophagus causing the discomfort but the acid is a vital part of your digestive system. With an already compromised digestive system, antacids are not the best solution to your heart burn. In addition, there is strong evidence that antacids prevent absorption of B vitamins through the intestines. B vitamins are the energy vitamins—need I say more? Do NOT use antacids.

Look for the cause of your eating problem; don't change the natural chemistry of your digestive system!

Pregnancy is a time to treat your body with respect and let it be the perfectly natural machine that it can be. Listen to your body. Accept that your body can give you the correct signals for what is needed. Do not put anything in your mouth that could alter your baby's perfect health. Take good care of you as well as the baby. You are a partnership—each affects the other. If you will recognize your heartburn as a warning that your diet and eating habits need reevaluating, I'm confident that you'll solve the problem.

I am addicted to fiery hot Mexican food. Every once in a while I crave it. I like it so hot that my lips, throat and tongue burn and tingle. You can imagine how my addiction and my pregnancies got along together! They didn't. About every three months I'd not be able to stand it any longer I would throw caution to the wind, have myself a feast and I would suffer all night long.

Usually you'll know, too, why you have indigestion. Try doing without that extra piece of dessert, or the second helping, or that hunk of delicious chocolate or whatever spicy foods are the cause of your heartburn. It is only for a few short months! My taste buds were happy when I broke training; my body wasn't—it's your choice what you do, but be aware—if you know what causes extreme discomfort, it might be best to avoid it for a few months.

> Your pregnant body won't let you cheat—not in bad posture or in bad eating. You hurt when you don't take care of yourself. Your body will let you know when you have broken the rules. It's not worth the discomfort or the risk to your baby.

Nausea of Pregnancy

I wish that none of you would ever experience this! It was an unpleasant part of my pregnancies—all five of them. I was lucky that I almost never had to vomit but only felt as though I might! My discomfort disappeared around the fourth month. Nausea in itself is not all that awful; it is just that it goes on and on, day after day until it becomes more of a depression than an illness. That explains how you can feel better when you get ready to go out to a fun event but are too sick to clean the kitchen after a meal. I remember having to choose between cooking dinner and having to endure the smells at a restaurant. Both were unappealing!

Nausea of pregnancy is like sea sickness. It is not that you feel so horribly ill but it's the hopelessness that there is no land to step on and get away from the rocking boat.

If you are unable to eat and can't keep food in your body, you must get medical help. Now! You cannot grow a healthy baby without food for both of you. There are medical solutions to this situation. Call your doctor. It is very different from what I am discussing here.

You will probably feel better if you eat small nibbles of food during the times of your nausea as well as keeping quiet while your body processes a small cracker or a few grapes. If you wake up feeling yucky keep a small snack of whole wheat crackers or a banana or something appealing to you and have a few nibbles before you even move out of bed.

Although food is unappealing, you must maintain a proper balanced diet. Small meals more frequently seems to help. Bites of fruit every hour keeps your blood sugar in a normal level as long as you will also eat protein at meals. Usually this problem works itself out rather quickly … I hope so, for both you and your baby!

Rhondda's Tip

Most discomforts of pregnancy are mild. Most likely, you'll realize that you need to change a bad habit or two. Certainly, that is possible to do. If you have a problem that you can't control, do not hesitate to call your health care provider for help and advice.

Chapter 10

Eating For Two ... or More?

You need to become extremely diet conscious now that you are pregnant. An interest in eating correctly is important to your health, your baby's health, your energy, figure and general happiness. Your primary concern is protein. That's the stuff of which bodies are made and you are making a new body in your uterus. If you will eat a well-balanced diet of protein, carbohydrates and fats you will have a healthy strong baby. Also you will look and feel better and your energy level will remain high.

Medical opinion about weight gain during pregnancy has gone through many changes during my lifetime. If you gain too much weight, it becomes a weight problem for you, but if you do not gain enough weight, you could damage your baby. Make sure that you have extra protein and well-balanced nutrition. Do not restrict anything but eat whole foods with lots of variety. Fresh fruit and vegetables and non-processed food will keep you healthy. Fast food is less likely to be the best choice but of course, most moms-to-be resort to it sometimes. My advice: don't make a habit of it, especially when pregnant.

There is conclusive evidence that alcohol and smoking are very harmful to a growing fetus. Please consider this seriously and commit to the health of your baby rather than your own unhealthy desires. Don't drink or smoke during pregnancy! As a matter of fact, it would be the best for the baby if you could cleanse your body of these poisons before you became pregnant. It is probably too late to tell you that now! But you now know it for future reference!

You may have to change your eating habits completely to become a well-nourished, healthy person, and now is a good time, while you are so conscious of your body and your baby. You do not have to eat three meals a day. Six may be much better for you. Throw out all the old ideas and start fresh!

Eating well can be a challenge but it can be such fun planning and preparing food. The food groups have changed over the years but this is the way I think of them: Proteins, Carbohydrates and Fats. All three are necessary to your health.

Proteins

The easiest protein comes from animal sources—meat, fish, chicken, eggs, cheese and milk. Most vegetables do have some protein content and seeds, grains and nuts are good sources. However, many vegetable proteins do not have all the essential amino acids and cannot be used properly in your body as builders unless you supply the missing amino acids to make a complete protein that can be used in the body as a building block. So when you use vegetables for your source of protein, you need to put the correct combinations together.

Beans and Boston brown bread give you complete protein. Peanut butter with milk makes a complete protein available for your body to use. Always use non-hydrogenated peanut butter or the protein is not available at all. Macaroni and cheese pair together to become a complete protein. So it becomes a bit more time consuming and takes more planning to be a vegetarian, especially in pregnancy when nutrition is so very important.

Many of the typical native dishes have been put together with this good common sense. Mexicans eat beans with corn tortillas. The Italians use pasta, cheese and tomatoes with olives. Germans have rich dark whole grain bread which is eaten with everything. The Chinese use a large variety of vegetables and soy beans. Soy beans are the best single source of vegetable protein. Native dishes are often very healthy and good for you. Amazing that these good-for-you recipes were put together without the use of nutritional guides!

Below is is a very simple, general guide to a well-balanced daily diet during pregnancy:

Proteins

Meat, fish, seeds, Grains, nuts, tofu, Beans, cheese, soy	Two servings per day.
Eggs	Two a day. This may conflict with some advice you will get, but egg is probably the most perfect protein you can eat and is a very good source of iron.
Milk	One quart a day (four cups.) The cheapest, easiest source of protein and calcium, which is necessary for the baby's bone development and nerve cells.

Carbohydrates—Simple and Complex

This seems to be the most confusing diet group for most of us. That is because there are simple carbs that are absorbed directly from the stomach into the blood stream. This is good for instant energy. Orange juice or any sugar drinks are examples. This raises the blood sugar to a high level. The brain does not like to have the blood sugar too high so it tells the pancreas to send insulin into the blood to carry the sugar to be stored for a time when it is needed and somehow it is stored as fat! I find it very complicated but ingenious!

Then there are the complex carbs which take more time and effort to break into useable blood sugar and are released into the blood more slowly and continuously. However, if the blood sugar gets too high the complex carbs, too, will be sent off to be stored as fat cells for a rainy day or for a time of starvation. Less insulin will be needed to take care of the complex carbs because it takes longer to digest and the blood sugar levels will not spike as severely.

For food to be used in the body it must be turned into sugar to be carried in the blood to the cells. Protein takes a longer time to be turned into blood sugar and so it is important in your diet to give a slow continuous supply to the body. I use the word "sugar" loosely here! I am trying to make the point clear that there is not good blood sugar or bad blood sugar but it is the way the body uses it. The system is perfect. Our bodies are amazing!

However, too many simple carbohydrates over use the pancreas and we have a disease of diabetes to show what can happen. Too much food, more than the body needs, also over uses the body's well planned endocrine system and compromises your health. Treat your body with respect and you will be rewarded by feeling well.

Simple Carbohydrates are: Juices, sugar drinks, pastries, sweets, chocolate and doughnuts.

Fruit juices are also simple carbs whereas fruits eaten as a fruit are somewhat more complex carbohydrates. Don't skip fruits—they are a necessary food group for the nutritive value.

When it comes to vegetables, you will learn that some are less complex than others.

The more calories there are in veggies, the more easily the starch is turned to sugar and that would make them a simpler carbohydrate.

As with fruits, vegetables are also a necessary food group.

Total fruits and vegetables to be eaten each day for a healthy diet are 7 to 11 servings per day. A general rule on this is the more color, the higher the nutritional value. Most of our vitamins and minerals come from this group. Lots of variety is important. You need to have at least one citrus fruit and one green leafy vegetable each day.

You can never eat too much as long as you have a good variety. I have seen toddlers turn yellow from too many carrots! Come on, moms, you can do better than too many carrots. Our choices are abundant and available!

Carbohydrates

Vegetables

At least one green leafy vegetable each day and a yellow, green or red vegetable each day. A general rule on veggies is that the more color, the more nutritional value.

Starchy vegetables

Potatoes, rice, corn, lentils, beans
More calories than vegetables above
Starch takes longer to digest than sugar but they are both carbohydrates.

Fruit

At least one citrus fruit each day— orange, grapefruit, or lemon—plus other fruits.

Total Fruits and Vegetables need to total at least 7-11 servings per day.
The greater the number and variety of servings of fruits and vegetables, the better!

Vegetables and fruits provide a wide assortment of vitamins and minerals for general health, and the more variety, the more of these nutrients you will be providing for your body. Fruits and vegetables are also the best source of carbohydrates in a well-balanced diet. They provide nature's unrefined sugars and starches, whereas white sugar, candy, and soft drinks are carbohydrates with no real food value—only calories. If you eat well, you will not have a craving for such "empty" calories. However, even empty calories *will* give your body energy!

Cereals and Bread … Are They a Carbohydrate or a Protein?

It is a combination of both so it can be a separate category! You need it for good health so:

> One serving each a day of whole-grain cereal as well as
> bread made from whole-grain flour … two slices a day.

Bread and cereals do not mean cakes, cookies, doughnuts, and prepared refined breakfast foods. Generally, whole-grain, less refined foods will taste better, satisfy you more, give you more nutrients, and keep the calories down.

It is important that you gain enough weight to have a happy pregnancy and a healthy baby, but you do not have to change your own size by too many pounds. It's very hard to gain fifty or sixty pounds by eating sensibly and properly—it's possible, but not likely. Yet, it's better to gain weight than to eat a poor diet. Usually the pounds go on with pie, cake, cookies, doughnuts, candy, and whipped toppings—none of which are important, health-giving foods. Rarely do fruits, vegetables, whole grain breads, butter, eggs, fish, meat and milk create a fat person—you get too full to eat too much! The food is satisfying enough to keep you from overeating.

Oils and Fats

Fat is necessary in your diet for metabolism including the absorption of vitamins A, D, E and K. Actually fat is a necessary nutrient in your diet for the general functioning of your body but has been given a bad reputation recently. Fat does not make you fat. This does not mean that you should over eat fatty fried meat, oily gravies and margarine-laden bread—all of those would be damaged fats, altered, heated or man-made. A serving of natural undamaged vegetable oil used on a salad plus the natural fat in many foods, especially omega 3 fish oil would be sufficient for your needs.

Use Moderation for Healthy Eating

A meal that looks attractive is very often well-balanced. If you have different colors and shapes and consistencies of foods, you will usually be balancing the nutrients. Likewise, a variety from meal-to-meal and from day-to-day will help balance the nutritional content. Try to eat a different kind of meat each day during the week. Use meat substitutes for some meals—beans and cheese or fish. Try a different salad with each dinner. Prepare a new vegetable or one you seldom eat. Experiment with different greens—try tossing a salad with oil and vinegar and your own choice of spices.

Concoct, create, and try new things. Do not serve the same color, shape, or texture of vegetables at one time. Mostly, avoid serving the same old thing seven days a week! Day-to-day food planning can get very dull unless you make it fun. You will become invigorated and feel excited about meal preparation if you try some new foods. You are challenged in these nine months, and on into the future breastfeeding months, to eat the most nutritious food you can for the sake of your baby. Make it an adventure. Let meal planning be one of your specialties.

If you eat foods that are natural—that is, as close to their original form as possible—you will get more food value and will spend less money on food.

+ Buy whole potatoes rather than powdered mashed potatoes.

+ Buy fresh fruit and vegetables rather than frozen and frozen rather than canned fruits and veggies, for the best nutritional value.

Of course, home-grown vegetables are best, since they come directly from the garden to the table. If you've ever grown your own, you know that even the taste is better. That is not possible for most of us but you might try to use foods in season.

> The more processing used,
> the less nutritional value is available.
> Try to avoid altered food!

Whole-grain cereals are more health-giving than refined, sweetened dry cereals. Whole grains ground into flour are more nutritious than refined, bleached flours. Convenience foods are generally of low nutritional value and very high cost. I am generalizing, and there are exceptions to everything. Powdered milk is cheap, and its nutritional value is just fine! I'd still prefer mine fresh from the bottle! I've no interest in milking the cow, however!

We are all creatures of habit, and many things we eat just because we've always eaten them. I ask you to begin thinking carefully about your diet and toss out those unimportant foods for quality ones. If your doughnut for coffee break and chocolate bar before bed are more important to you than ten extra pounds, that is your choice; but don't leave out your daily orange and multiple servings of vegetables.

You are in for a great treat if you've never looked into the composition of foods until now. It is really exciting to see what foods contain. It's sometimes surprising that what you feel guilty about eating is really good for you. I remember a friend eating only the crusts of bread and not eating the center of the slice because it was not as good for her! The fact is that B vitamins are destroyed by heat so the crust is not as rich in vitamin B as the center of the slice. There you go, kids, cut off those offensive crusts! (Of course, if you're eating white bread, you're not getting much out of it anyway.) Find out what it has in it that's good for you, and you can justify eating it—maybe!

What I ask of each and every one of you is to become curious about what you eat. Look up the value of each thing you eat to find out whether it's good for you or not very important nutritionally. Become selective. Here is a time in your life when your eating habits directly affect another human being. Surely you care enough to provide the best possible chance of having a perfectly created baby.

Please don't misunderstand me ... I'm not asking you to become a fanatic about one style of eating or another. You can have a healthy, well-balanced diet from the supermarket; from eating vegetarian foods; growing your own crops organically; taking vitamin pills as supplements; eating wheat germ, liver and brewer's yeast till you get to like them; or having to stick to a medically recommended diet.

A Word About Salt … Salt to Taste!

Salt is necessary for a healthy pregnancy and a healthy baby.

Your body cannot function without salt. During pregnancy the amniotic fluid must be constantly produced and refreshed so extra salt is used. Who came up with the idea that in pregnancy you should restrict salt? Dr. Thomas Brewer was teaching that salt was necessary for healthy babies years ago but found it hard to convince the medical profession. Gail Brewer has carried on since his death advocating for babies. Check out the website *www.BlueRibbonBaby.com*. You will get all the information you need about nutrition in pregnancy. Dr. Brewer developed a healthy diet and the research to prove its effectiveness. It is very detailed and complete. You will find it useful.

Vitamins and You

The amazing thing about nutrition is the amount of new information being found every day from scientific research. What I learned in Nursing School has been added to with huge changes. Everyone was taught the Food Groups in grade school and by high school, they were revised. Decades later, the whole food pyramid has morphed into something totally unfamiliar. New vitamins are being discovered and added to our nutrients as necessary for our wellbeing.

One of the "ahas" in the last few years is that Vitamin D is being blocked from our bodies with sunblock products. Depending upon where you live (such as the southern belt vs. the northern belt of the United States, just the mere positioning of your state will affect the amount of rays that naturally come from the sun. And— "Oh, by the way,"—the experts are now saying that was an insufficient amount of Vitamin D from the sun in the first place—that we all need a supplement for it! Vitamin D is the "newest cure everything vitamin" as I write! During pregnancy a smart mother-to-be makes sure that she gets balanced nutrition for both her and her baby. Just don't overdo it, thinking that more is better. What you take in; so does your baby.

> Caution: don't be surprised when the vitamin gurus stake their claim for another vitamin of the month/year. The point here is to be alert—take care of you and your baby with the best information that you can get—it all starts with the basic diet mentioned above.

The media has news on nutrition constantly! So please take what I am telling you about this subject as a capsule in time from me. Some of what I have said may be wrong already! I am definitely not a licensed nutritional expert but I do keep changing and adding to my information about eating well and staying healthy. It's in my pedigree to do so. My father lived to be 100, my mother 97. With my genes, it is important that I try to keep my health!

Do your own thing with food, but make sure you give your body adequate protein, carbohydrates, and fats, plus all the vitamins and minerals so essential for good health. I have given you general ideas only. Please find a good reference on nutrition, I recommend Dr. Brewer, and make sure you follow it.

Remember: you are responsible for the health of you *and* your baby.

Now that nutrition is so vital to a healthy baby, keep away from all the ideas that have been popular about low fat and no salt.

You need them in natural foods as they exist in nature. Nothing refined or stripped of one thing or another. Eat butter, whole milk and salt to taste along with all real food that dieting programs have made you believe to be bad for you.

One more thing: My apologies to the knowledgeable nutrition experts who are reading this. I have greatly oversimplified and exaggerated to make my points. I am not an expert and I do not intend this to be a complete nutritional guide. Please use the internet to explore the possibilities of diet and health.

I have my favorite gurus and I am sure you have yours. Let's have conversations and sharing on my website,

www.NaturalChildbirthExercises.com

Rhondda's Tip

It is vital that you have good nutrition, as the size and health of your baby depend on what you eat each day. Bad eating habits could cause low-birth-weight babies, infection-prone babies, and even brain-damaged babies. Your diet is important for you as well as the baby: to prevent anemia; to prevent toxemia of pregnancy (a disease of late pregnancy that can lead to all kinds of complications); to protect you from severe infections; and to protect you from miscarriage.

Chapter 11

Veins, Legs, Feet and Cramps ... Oh My!

By the time you are in the middle of your pregnancy, your feet and legs may be expressing some discomfort with your added weight and the new way you may be walking as you balance your girth.

Even without a pregnancy, the mother of other small children is feeling rather "worn out" by the end of a busy, chasing day. Adding a pregnancy can lead to a tsunami of fatigue.

However, the great majority of women feel fantastic these middle months. With all the skills you've been learning along with your "I'm feeling good" attitude, let's discuss some new postures and movements for a healthier, happier and more comfortable pregnancy that focus on your feet and legs.

Varicose Veins

Do you understand what varicose veins are? It is a subject we should discuss, since the occurrence of them, is higher in women than in men, and the incidence in women increases with pregnancy.

Obvious varicose veins are ugly, tortuous, swollen blue veins that show on your legs—especially behind the knees. Sometimes there is nothing visible on the legs because it is the deep veins that have the problem.

The degree of obviousness has no correlation with the symptoms produced. Some legs with obvious blue veins will cause no symptoms and another person who shows no varicose veins will have severe discomfort. Symptoms commonly are aching, tense legs with an itching or burning sensation of the skin, often accompanied by cramping of the calf muscle.

Varicose veins are aggravated by pregnancy for two reasons. First, the blood volume increases during pregnancy, causing an added burden to the circulatory system. Secondly, the main vessels of circulation to the legs run inside the pelvis, where the enlarging uterus is creating pressure. Since the pelvis is a bony structure, it can cause a constriction of those arteries and veins.

Your main concern is to maintain a good blood supply to the uterus and therefore your baby. Blood supply to the kidneys is also a major concern. Arterial blood has the advantage of working with gravity but venous blood must fight an uphill battle. Further, the veins are not nearly as flexible and elastic as arteries (evolution made a small error there!).

The veins do have valves which help prevent the backward flow of blood and the muscle tension of the legs helps keep blood moving. However, that extra slowdown, as the veins are slightly compressed by the pressure of the uterus in the pelvis, can be the final straw. There begins a build-up of blood in the veins of the legs and instead of a fast-running river of blood, you have some "puddles and lakes" here and there. This compromises the elasticity of the walls of the veins and damages the valve system, so that backflow of the blood occurs, making the progress of venous flow toward the heart even more arduous. You can have swelling of the legs and feet and severe aching of legs. The danger of infection in a vein (phlebitis) is a possibility, and ulceration of skin can also occur. However this would be very unusual in a young pregnant woman!

Is this enough to convince you that prevention is vitally important? Heredity is an added contributing factor to this whole picture. If your mother or father has varicose veins, your chances of the same are very high. Prevention is very important.

It should be mentioned that anything wrapped tightly around your legs will inhibit the proper flow of blood, and could be a factor in causing varicose veins. Tight knee-highs and socks will do your veins no favors. Avoid them.

Support hose and elastic stockings, on the other hand, may bring comfort and relief to you who already suffer from painful legs. You can order special elastic stockings made to measure for you. That will make you much more comfortable, but you can help maintain good circulation with the postures and exercises that are explained in Leg Elevation Exercise.

Remember that pregnancy does aggravate the condition, so that after the baby is born you will have less trouble or no trouble, depending upon the condition of your veins. Work hard at these circulation exercises even though you have no apparent signs of varicose veins. Small breaks in the capillaries of the skin are not varicose veins but are an indication of some distress and a good warning to you.

Leg Cramps

A possible annoying complaint of pregnancy is leg cramps, particularly in the calf muscle. It is easily treated. Simply point your heel as you stretch your leg out straight. In fact, the cramp can be avoided as soon as you feel the crampiness beginning. Here's how: you pull your toes toward your face—that is, point your heel. If, however, you are asleep and by the time you've wakened, the cramp or "charley horse" is well established then I advise standing, full weight, on the offending leg. You will need to walk a few steps to get your muscles "untangled" and back working again.

You can give yourself a muscle spasm by pointing your toe—avoid doing that. Your <u>heel</u> is the correct body part to point!

If you have many leg cramps, tell your health care provider. He or she may have you change your diet or advise a vitamin, an example is CoQ10 that will help. Another possible solution is the mineral supplement of calcium and magnesium.

Also, remember; point your heel, not your toe!

Leg Exercises that Make a Difference

The following exercises are offered with circulation of the lower extremities in mind. Use them faithfully and you may virtually defy heredity. Leg elevation is really a treat so be sure to get the proper equipment ready and keep it handy.

One good way to elevate your lower body is by raising the foot of your bed with three or four bricks. Your spouse may not like the idea at first, but after a few days he may find that he is more rested and has lost that "woody" feeling in his legs, too. Men can have the same problem, even without a uterus!

Keep Your Circulation Moving

Foot Circles and Leg Stretches are easy, fast, and will get your sluggish circulation speeded up. Leg Elevation will be helpful and feels great. Don't forget that hands-and-knees Pelvic Rock is one of the most important ways of eliminating pelvic pressure on those veins and getting the blood pushed through your circulatory system. I told you that it would be a cure-all. "When in doubt, do some Pelvic Rocks" is my motto.

Leg Elevation

Since varicose veins are a constant threat during pregnancy and even though the problem lessens after the birth, the probability of some vein damage stays with you. So the more you can do to prevent any vein damage during pregnancy, the better off you are for life.

Sometimes varicose veins will occur in the perineum, especially in the vaginal area. A symptom of this condition is pain and pressure in the perineum immediately upon getting out of bed in the morning. It is caused by the rush of blood to the area. You should find pelvic rocks on hands and knees helpful at this time, though leg elevation is the best relief and prevention position.

On-your-back sleepers, beware: It is absolutely not good for you to lie on your back during pregnancy. It is all about the weight of the baby on those important blood vessels. If you like to sleep on your back, reread all that I have said about blood supply to your baby. As your uterus grows you will become very uncomfortable, so even you confirmed back sleepers will manage to give up your habit with no trouble.

As for these postures and exercises on your back:

Hold these postures for no more than 10 minutes at a time!

Do lots of leg elevations to try to prevent any more damage to the veins. Lying on your back can be harmful, as I have stressed again and again! Therefore, do your leg elevation for short periods of time only!

Ten minutes is maximum! Although you are lying on your back in what amounts to an inverted contour position, the reverse tilt of your pelvis virtually eliminates pressure. It feels so good that you may have to watch the clock to avoid staying in the posture too long. The gentle slope of the lower part of your body helps gravity return your blood efficiently to the heart.

Preparation:

The idea is simple. You tip your head down and your legs up to allow the blood in the lower half of your body to flow back toward the heart.

The equipment can be simple, too. An inclined plane and two pillows are all you need. If you own a slant board, use it. Tilt the bottom of it up about twelve inches, put a pillow under your knees, and you are set. Make it comfortable.

A contour chair or folding beach chair will do. Put your legs up the backrest and your head down. You may need a pillow under your lower back to be comfortable, and be sure that the backs of the knees are supported comfortably with a pillow. If too much contortion is required, don't use it! Find a simpler solution.

An ordinary kitchen chair can be used with extra pillows, blankets or some good padding, as I show on the next page.

You can make a slant board with a piece of wood as long and as wide as you are. You may be able to find a good piece of plywood in your garage—or go to the lumberyard. Wrap a blanket around the board and tie it on so that it won't slip—or upholster it with foam rubber and a fabric you like. The whole thing can be done rather inexpensively and you will not have to search for the makings every time you do the elevation. Prop up one end of the board on several bricks or the second step of your stairway. Put a pillow under your knees and you will feel fantastic.

If you use a chair as I have used, you'll need extra pillows to elevate your hips.

If your legs and feet begin to "fall asleep," be sure to slide off the slant board onto the floor or bed, assuming a side-lying relaxation position. When you get up, be sure to do it slowly to avoid the dizziness that often happens when rising from a prone position in pregnancy. Gravity helps the blood flow down in your body and leaves your head too quickly. Adjustment only takes a few seconds. A few pelvic rocks will solve the dizziness.

Leg Elevation Position

Now that you have your chair and pillows arranged, place yourself into the position as shown.

HOW:

+ Your head is lower than your heels.

+ Your hips are elevated above your heart so that you can feel the uterus pulled up and out of the pelvis.

+ Your knees are supported on a pillow in a slightly flexed, relaxed position.

+ As the blood rushes to the upper part of your body (which is now lowered), you may feel hot and flushed for a bit and your breathing may be "puffy."

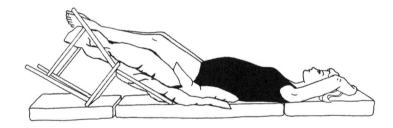

Bonus Exercises

While in this position, there are other exercises you can do that will enhance your leg circulation and help prevent varicose veins. Use them, you'll like them.

Leg Elevation Exercises

HOW:

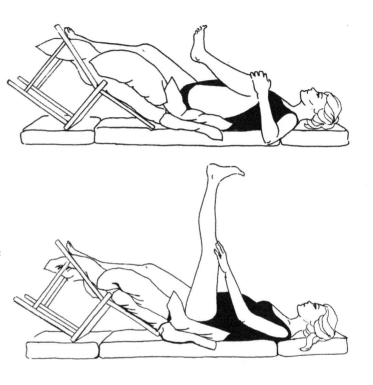

1. Bend one knee up toward your chest.

2. Straighten that leg up in the air with your heel pointed. (Do not point your toe or you may get a leg cramp.)

3. Lower the leg slowly to its original position, keeping your heel pointed.

4. Relax your leg completely and be sure the knee is partially flexed and slightly turned out.

5. Repeat with other leg.

6. Repeat each leg several times. A set of 8 on each leg is a good amount.

WHERE:

In your "already set up" Leg Elevation Position—with your head lower than your heels, a pillow under your lower back, and another under your knees to loosen them. It should be a handy spot so you are encouraged to get into this position often. Have the phone nearby and ignore the doorbell. Getting up quickly is not advisable.

WHEN:

If you have varicose veins already, you will want to do this posture very often. Sometimes doctors recommend that you put your feet up ten minutes out of each hour. I repeat, since you will be on your back, 10 minutes an hour would be the maximum amount of time to spend in this position.

Foot Circles Exercises

This is another good exercise to help minimize varicose veins and it makes you feel better and more energetic, too.

By forcing the circulation of blood through your legs, you create an efficient exchange of nutrients and wastes to and from the tissues.

It is better than a walk because the uterus does not become hammered into the pelvis to create pressure, as happens with walking. The good effects of walking when pregnant are somewhat cancelled by the pressure created in the pelvis. So we offer foot circles as an alternative!

HOW:

1. Sit on the floor, leaning back against a pillow or against your sofa with your right knee bent.

2. Rest your left ankle on your right knee.

3. Do a series of nine circles to the outside of your foot (clockwise).

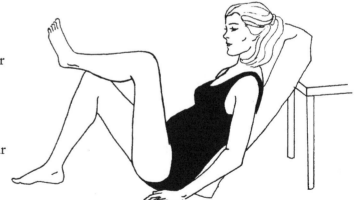

4. When you've finished nine circles, your toes are pointing up. Then relax your foot and shake out your whole leg, so that any muscle crampiness is released.

5. Do the same thing with the right ankle resting on the left knee, making counterclockwise circles.

6. Now enjoy the good feeling in your legs and feet.

Think of tracing the face of a clock with your big toe. Start with your big toe pointing straight up to an imaginary twelve o'clock. Then your toes point to three o'clock, six o'clock, nine o'clock, and then twelve o'clock again. Do three quarter circles, three half circles, three whole circles, all clockwise. Do the opposite with the left foot—go counterclockwise.

Added benefit: This will help strengthen the arch in your foot so that you need not be flat-footed with pregnancy.

WHERE:

Anywhere that you can relax and get into position you can do foot circles. It's very comfortable to lean against your husband while you do this.

WHEN:

Do this anytime your legs feel tired. It is especially indicated if you've not rested sufficiently during the day. You can't control every day the way you'd like, so sometimes a revitalizing exercise is the perfect antidote. It is particularly useful when you have been busy most of the day and have not done enough pelvic rocks (except the standing type which I hope you were able to fit in.)

Let's say you arrive home tired. Before dinner is a perfect time for foot circles! You could do some hands-and-knees pelvic rocks, too, maybe take an extra five minutes to just relax. If your spouse is around, ask him to check your relaxation. Now you can go about your normal routine and the evening will proceed more smoothly because you feel better. Your pregnancy will be so much easier and more pleasant if you will take care of your body as the primary concern of the family.

It's easy to think, "I don't have time to do all these things," but what you are saying is, "I don't think it's important enough to take time." You are important and so is your baby in utero, which makes you twice as important.

Leg Stretches—Flexing and Extending Ankles and Knees

Not only will leg stretches stimulate circulation in your legs; they will also strengthen your leg muscles and make it easier to carry those extra pounds caused by your growing baby. You may even develop a more shapely leg! You will be carrying your child for at least a year after he is born, too, so let's get ready now. If you wear high heels, this exercise will help stretch your Achilles tendon, which may have become shortened over the years. It is a good idea, pregnant or not, to vary the type of heel you wear.

Walking or running barefoot in sand is supposed to be the best exercise for your legs and feet. Sand moves under your feet as you walk to provide a workout for your muscles. Hard floors or cement sidewalks do not "move." Since running barefoot in the sand is not possible for all of us, I've included these easy leg stretches.

HOW:

1. From a tailor sit position, stretch one or both legs away from you at an angle, supporting yourself with your hands.

2. Extend your toes away from you while stretching your leg out straight.

3. Pull your toes toward your body and raise your knee at thesame time. The heel will rotate but for maximum effect it should not move from its position. You can do legs separately or together until you feel comfortable. Resume your tailor sitting.

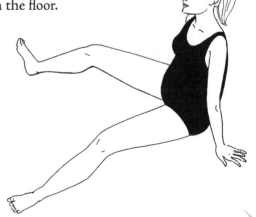

WHERE:

These Leg Stretches can be done anywhere you are tailor sitting on the floor.

WHEN:

They are especially useful when you are involved in an activity and sitting in the tailor sit position. If you feel the need to move but do not wish to interrupt your writing or reading—or simply do not have the energy to move around—this accomplishes the same thing.

Rhondda's Tip

So often mothers feel overworked and are over-busy. Think of this: it's a gift to your family, and yourself, to take some time—whether it's 15 or 60 minutes—to keep your body healthy and comfortable.

Chapter 12

Getting Ready for Proper Pushing

The "middle trimester" is the name given to the fourth, fifth and sixth months. When you are in your fifth month, the baby is about ten inches long and weighs about one pound. He's become a hefty cantaloupe in size with plenty of room to stretch and kick. He has hair, his teeth have begun to form and his bones would show on x-ray. You are feeling the gymnastics that he can perform!

You are now about halfway into your pregnancy and definitely showing. It's a good time for comparing sizes with the other pregnant women. There are great discrepancies between tummy sizes. Some of you look near term, others barely show.

All inhibitions are lost among you as you talk about your pregnancies with your friends. The differences in your lives are ignored as you discuss the similarities of your pregnancies and contemplate being mothers. For mothers-to-be, pregnancy is a great leveler and a common bond surfaces.

Confidence at this time is very high. If you are in a Childbirth class, it's not uncommon for a class member to be assured enough to take over temporarily, relating her experiences or her point of view. Those who've had babies before are especially eager to tell the others "how it is." This is a help, as experiences shared with others offer variety and bring up related matters that might never have surfaced otherwise. If you do not have a class to attend, I hope you can find some other support group with women who are eager to share their pregnancy experiences.

You have now had time to become proficient at the basic exercises.

Let's review:
+ Tailor sitting is done easily and often.
+ Abdominal breathing is by no means perfect, but has become easy.
+ Relaxing needs more work but you are feeling good about it.
+ Pelvic rock has become your best friend and you use it more and more often.

This trimester is the most comfortable period of pregnancy. Nausea is usually gone, or at least greatly improved. People talk about your "glow" … you look great. The pregnant uterus is big enough to be riding up and out of the pelvis but not heavy enough to be causing much pressure. Your mental outlook is generally superb. You are enjoying becoming a mother.

Getting Ready for Pushing and Giving Birth

With your expanding girth, it's time to think about the actual process of giving birth to your baby. You will need to begin practicing breath holding for the all-important pushing phase which is the second stage of labor. You also need to learn the ultimate position for giving birth. You learned to squat … now you need to put that into a position that is also used for the pushing stage of labor.

You are becoming proficient at abdominal breathing. Now let's learn the breathing that will make a difference for your second-stage labor. First let me present my "nutshell" review of instructions for Natural Childbirth.

Natural Childbirth in a Nutshell

1. **In the First Stage of labor**, use abdominal breathing and complete relaxation with each contraction.

2. **In the Second Stage of labor**, take complete, full breaths with each contraction and push as hard as you can while holding your breath.

Breath Holding

It is important that you have a big breath to be able to push properly. Only with full lungs can you push down adequately with your diaphragm. The more usable oxygen you have in your lungs, the longer you can hold your breath and push. The longer you can push without having to replenish your breath, the sooner you will give birth!

However, if you are trying to push after your breath has been used up it will not be working for you. Take a breath when you need more oxygen. That is the only way your pushing will be effective.

Each time you stop pushing to take a breath, the baby slips back in the birth canal. As you reapply the pressure of pushing, the baby descends and forces open the birth canal. Each push is a step forward; when you relax it's a small step back. This is truly hard work. Your body needs enormous amounts of oxygen … good, big breaths are necessary for effective pushing.

Learning now to breathe properly for the second stage will greatly improve your efficiency and reduce the time you are in labor.

The position for pushing is very important, too. In a squat position with chin on chest, all your energy is directed toward the baby, helping push the baby through the birth canal. It's as though your back is a bowstring pulled back as far as it will go. The baby is the arrow! The energy of the bowstring gives the impetus to the arrow. You might not be on your feet in a squat, though that would be ideal, but rather tilted into a forty-five-degree angle, with your arms pulling your legs back, elbows up and out. You will be half sitting, with your husband supporting your shoulders.

As though that is not enough to concentrate on, there is one more thing to remember—relax that baby door, the Kegel muscle. In this position, you can push your baby into the world efficiently and quickly.

HOW:

Tailor sitting posture seems best for practicing this breathing, but whatever position is comfortable for you is fine. The actual position that is used in labor—contour—may be uncomfortable during late pregnancy because the baby is so high up in the abdomen, making breathing very difficult as he pushes into your lungs. In second-stage labor, however, the baby has descended very low into the pelvis and in fact is at least partly in the birth canal, so there is plenty of space for the lungs to work properly.

To practice:

1. Sit comfortably in a Tailor position.

2. Take a very large breath, until your lungs feel expanded. Exhale fully.

3. Repeat. You have now taken two large breaths, exhaling each completely.

4. Take another full, deep breath and hold.

5. Hold as long as the breath lasts—about forty seconds seems a good practice time. (As Dr. Bradley said, "No need for heroics!")

6. When you've held as long as is comfortable, exhale fully.

In Labor:

- *Pull knees back*

- *Keep elbows up and out*

- *Chin on chest*

Take the first 2 breaths and blow them out. As you take your third breath, you will also be drawing your knees toward your shoulders and pulling your legs back with your hands, elbows up and out. As you begin holding your breath you'll put your chin to your chest and bear down on the baby with strong, steady pushing.

You will be nearly in a squat position, which is the most efficient position for giving birth. Keep your elbows out, pulling your knees back. Do not lift your tailbone off the bed. You want to push the baby downhill, not uphill. When you have held your breath and pushed as long as is effective, lift your chin off your chest, exhale completely and take another big breath, chin on chest and keep pushing. As long as there is a contraction going on, you keep pushing.

If you need to take a breath several times, do it. When the pushing contraction is over, relax and wait for the next. This is extremely hard work but it is also the only way to feel good during a pushing contraction! You will become unaware of the pressure and discomfort as you push hard.

If you feel pain you may not be pushing correctly or hard enough.

You must work with your body. There is nothing to be gained in pushing when the uterus is not in a contraction. Natural Childbirth is simply working with your body when it needs help and staying out of its way when the body does not need any help. You see how simple this is?

First Stage of Labor: Relax to stay out of the way of your uterus as it contracts. You have no conscious control over the muscles of the cervix which must stretch to open with the pressure of the baby's head. Your job is to relax to stay out of the way of your body. It is the body's natural response to the birth process. You interfere if you do anything but relax during a contraction.

Second Stage of Labor: When the uterus contracts you work with it by pushing. As long as there is a contraction, you push. You do have control of muscles that help get the baby through the birth canal, which is your vagina. The uterus no longer has the full body of your baby completely within it. Pushing helps during a contraction! It also takes away the pain. Push through the pain.

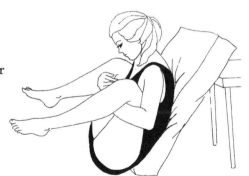

WHERE and WHEN:

During labor, you will use this breathing whenever and wherever you are when you receive that unmistakable urge to push!

Meanwhile, practice daily to improve your breath-holding ability. Have your husband rehearse with you since he'll undoubtedly hold his breath during your pushes in labor anyway. It's automatic—have you ever tried to breathe normally while watching someone else hold his or her breath? It will also give your husband experience in coaching for this final step of labor.

Practice the breath holding <u>only</u>. Practicing pushing will only contribute to hemorrhoids and is unnecessary, as those muscles are kept strong by your natural body functions, that is, in bowel elimination.

With your new breathing skills and your "I'm feeling good" attitude, let's learn one more thing that will make your pushing better and easier. That means a quicker and more comfortable pushing stage of labor as well as being more comfortable after the baby is in your arms.

Butterfly—or Legs Apart Exercises

This will strengthen the legs-apart muscles, or abductors. They are weaker than the muscles that pull your legs together (the adductors) … and holding your legs apart is very important—especially during second-stage labor. Your abductors need added strength.

Not only do you need your legs apart during a push, but between pushes, too, because the baby is low in the birth canal at this time. If your muscles have been completely fatigued with the effort to keep your legs apart during second stage, you may not have enough strength left to support you when you are ready to stand!
Even if you don't walk immediately, you may have trembling, weak legs for several days if you have not prepared.

HOW:

Sit in contour position with knees drawn up and feet together on the floor. Have your husband, partner or coach put their hands on the outside of each of your knees and exert gentle pressure as you push your knees apart as far as they will go. You may change your feet so that the soles are together—it's more comfortable.

Bring your knees back together (with no pressure against them) and repeat twice more, with slightly increased pressure each time you spread your knees apart (like a butterfly's wings).

Warnings about your coach:

It is possible to have more strength in their arms than you do in your legs. That will do you no good if you can't practice to build up these muscles so you must teach the rules for this game! Some will think that if three times is good, three hundred is better. Not so here. Stiff abductor muscles make every movement painful. Tell your coach to only do it three times! Also, this muscle, overbuilt, is not pretty, nor is it our objective to have a bulging muscle … just a stronger one. Do not put pressure on your knees as you return your legs to the upright, beginning position. This would strengthen the already much stronger adductors—nullifying what we're trying to accomplish.

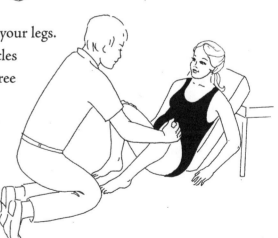

And do not let anyone push your knees to the floor as you are spread apart. Ouch!

You do not believe your coach will do any of these things to you, do you? Believe me I have not made them up. They are experiences class members have told me about repeatedly—so I warn you in advance.

WHERE and WHEN:

Wherever and whenever the two of you decide and have the energy to practice. It only takes a few minutes to do three of these once a day. Getting organized to do it will take more time than doing it! It is worth it as it will have a significant effect on your leg strength post birth.

Rhondda's Tip

Remember—when you have a big breath, you are able to push properly in labor. The more usable oxygen you have in your lungs, the longer you can hold your breath and push. Be sure to take breaths as needed! The more oxygen you have to make your push effective, the sooner you will give birth. Your reward!

Chapter 13

Planning for Breastfeeding

Somewhere around the sixth month, you really feel you have a baby coming—he has made his presence well known with his internal kicks and stretches. If you haven't thought about it, or decided, I've found that this is usually a good time to begin thinking about whether you will breast feed or bottle feed your baby. As you end the second trimester, your baby is over a foot in length and weighs a few pounds. If photos are taken of you, don't be surprised to note that you unconsciously embrace your growing belly.

A new feeling is noted by this time. For some, the glow that surfaced after morning sickness begins to fade a bit. Six months have gone by rather speedily, all agree—but almost unanimously, most wish it could hurry to full term. The weight of the baby sometimes becomes a burden now. It is getting to be more difficult to continue some activities. For the athlete—it's common to have many of the more strenuous activities toned down—the skier steps away from the extreme slopes; the bowler finds the lanes a bit challenging; the equestrian stops her galloping mounts; and the marathoner moves into walking. That bulging tummy simply gets in the way!

It's a good time to think about preparing yourself mentally and physically for breastfeeding.

Breastfeeding

I always assume that anyone who is going to have Natural Childbirth is going to breastfeed her baby ... The first nine months were natural; the second nine-month period should follow the same philosophy.

Breastfeeding is the most normal, natural, healthful, and satisfying method of feeding—not to mention the easiest and most economical! Once breastfeeding is established, it is the perfect supply-meets-demand system. The baby's need for milk automatically triggers the breast to produce the required amount. If the nutritional needs of the baby increase, he will nurse more often and suck longer and the breast will step up production of milk. It is a magnificent system, but of course, being human, we can throw it out of order.

> Studies show that allergies can be prevented by breastfeeding as well as a late introduction of other foods (four to six months). There are many studies which show that breastfeeding prolongs babies' natural immunity to infections.

If everyone in your family and most of your friends nursed their babies, it is a comfortable idea to you and will be easy. If this is totally unusual to you, it will make it harder. The insecurity of being one of the few people you know who have ever breastfed a baby can be enough to put problems in your way. Many of you have never known anyone who breastfed. You think breastfeeding is something that "primitives" do. Or perhaps the only woman you ever knew who did nurse her baby was someone you did not like. Does your *husband* want you to nurse his baby? How about your Mother-in-law or best friend? These and countless other factors may influence your decision to breastfeed and your ease in doing so.

First you must understand the facts about breastfeeding. Folklore and old wives' tales abound, but factual material is now in abundance, too, thanks to La Leche League International which publishes *The Womanly Art of Breast Feeding* and has created an audience for many other good books published on this subject.

The La Leche League's website, *www.LLLI.org,* is an excellent resource for ongoing articles, trouble-shooting and support. There are branches globally. To find one you near you, use the internet to find La Leche League in your city.

This organization has been a force for change in having breastfeeding acknowledged as "best for babies." It is and has been a very effective movement around the world as a group of mothers supporting each other in accepting and successfully achieving this natural system of feeding a baby.

It is a smart idea to attend La Leche League meetings if possible because they offer (1) a comprehensive course on the various aspects of breast-feeding and (2) companionship with other breastfeeding mothers. What you can learn in a discussion with other mothers is amazing! In fact, that is just how La Leche League began.

The "founding mothers" discussion of breast-feeding at a picnic turned into group discussion meetings and then blossomed into a huge international organization. Mothers sharing knowledge is the basis of each meeting. La Leche League fulfills another fundamental need: you may call your leader, who is an experienced breast-feeding mother with special training, anytime of the day or night with any problem you are having with your nursing baby. You can enter a chat room and talk with other moms that share their words and wisdom. Can you see what a beautiful situation that is? You have a friend and counselor as close as your telephone or computer.

With La Leche League so well set up to handle education for breastfeeding; it does make sense that we, who educate you for Natural Childbirth, wean you to breastfeeding experts to take over with the second aspect of becoming parents. Duplication of classes is a waste of time and effort, so if there is a local group, I would encourage you to join up and attend for information. Frequently, childbirth educators are also La Leche League leaders. I am a Charter Member in the Colorado Chapter with Mary Ann Kerwin, a Co-founding Mother of the original La Leche League International who moved to Denver. I was a LLLI Leader for many years as the organization flourished in Colorado.

If there is no group in your area, you can be instrumental in starting one. Check the web site and you will be surprised to find groups near you. At the very least, use the Le Leche League's cornerstone book, *The Womanly Art of Breastfeeding* as your operation manual. Some of you may reject the "meeting" idea, so it is all in print for you!

Now that I have introduced you to the value of the La Leche League, let me give you some of the highlights of breastfeeding that I've learned with breastfeeding five children and working with thousands of women.

Mother's milk is the natural food for your baby. In these days of dispute over what nutrients are or are not in foods, and what is or is not required, it is very comforting not to have to convert cow's milk into something one hopes is suitable for a human infant. If you eat as well as you know how, your milk will have in it at least everything that your body can supply. Obviously, your good nutrition is important.

When you breastfeed, the baby's milk is always ready. In the middle of the night this is especially pleasant. If your baby sleeps in your room, it's just a few steps away to change him and settle into a comfy chair, or even back to your warm bed.

I know, I know, some of you may be worried that you will roll over and suffocate your baby. Has it happened? Perhaps, but I have never heard of it! In my many years of working with new mothers, all have been alert in the care and feeding in those early weeks. (If you are taking any form of medication or drugs then it would not be a good idea.) Sometimes you both fall asleep and don't wake up until it's time for the next feeding, which is super easy—just turn over and put the baby on the other side.

If that idea does not appeal to you, the greatest effort you can put into a night feeding is donning slippers and robe, padding to the nursery, and putting yourself and baby into a rocking chair. In a family that's usually hectic with the activities of small children or busyness of any kind, these moments can be a peaceful communion between the two of you.

Nursing moms do want to be on alert if their baby reacts negatively to certain foods that the mother has eaten. Remember, what you eat can pass through your milk. Sometimes spicy foods, even garlic, can affect the baby. Most doctors are concerned about any drugs that a mother takes, as they too travel through your milk. When you were pregnant, you ate for two. Now that you are nursing, what you eat, drink and take will still affect the two of you.

Instant Readiness vs. Constant Pacifier

Instant readiness is important at times other than the middle of the night. Feeding is quickly available wherever you are. How easy it is to put baby to breast anytime the slightest bit of fussing begins.

Too easy, in fact, as you might be using yourself as a pacifier. You could have your baby snacking all day long and never settling down to a routine. It may discourage you from breastfeeding, too, if you seem to nurse continuously. However, when it is feeding time which is established by the baby and not by the clock, usually at three-hour intervals, you have the baby satisfied immediately. If it's "fussy time" for the baby, sometimes only Mommy can make him secure, and that's when your role as pacifier can be used and is such a relief!

Breastfeeding can be assisted with one arm, leaving the other free for making peanut butter sandwiches, holding a book as you read to your three-year-old, or just general loving of the other children.

A breastfeeding mother can take her baby with her anywhere very easily. A pediatric psychiatrist told me at a panel discussion on breastfeeding that she had taken a nursing baby to a formal banquet. One mother was featured in the *Denver Post*, riding her bicycle to the University of Denver with her baby on her back and taking the baby to classes. No bottles to carry! And the milk is always the perfect temperature.

The secret of all this "take the baby anywhere" is to have a blouse that allows breastfeeding without exposing yourself. No one minds seeing you in a bikini, but try showing any cleavage while breastfeeding your baby and you may face the *morality squad*. I cannot explain the rationale, but check out advice columns and you'll discover frequent entries on the subject—both pro and con. I found it particularly rewarding to nurse a baby in public with no one the wiser (a little game I played). I would occasionally get caught but it never seemed to offend anyone.

> Today, with clever clothing designed for nursing moms and many workplaces actually setting aside space for their employees who desire privacy, breast feeding your baby can be done without anyone the wiser.

Breastfeeding offers what a baby needs emotionally as well as nutritionally. Our Rienne is a good example. I "wore" her for months. She was either at the breast or on my hip. She was the third child in our family and we moved during that year so with all the confusion it is no wonder she clung to me. I began to worry about the dependent and clinging toddler I would have. I was her universe—she wanted nothing to do with anyone but me.

Nursing periods were gradually becoming slightly farther apart—and suddenly, with no other warning, she weaned herself at 13 months, as though she'd had a plan! As my milk supply did not have an on-off switch, I was indeed uncomfortable for a few days. She was completely happy with her "sippy" cup. Her need for breast feeding had apparently been satisfied and independence has always been a dominant factor in her personality ever since.

Give a breastfed baby what they want as they express that need. Trust the baby and yourself!

Get Back in Shape Faster

Breastfeeding has its physical rewards for the mother, too. It facilitates involution of the uterus, which returns to its normal size more quickly because the baby's sucking causes a simultaneous reflex contraction in the uterus. These are also known as after-birth "pains" which you now understand are just contractions. Nursing your baby while you are still on the delivery table can help the uterus to contract vigorously which helps control bleeding.

Dr. Bradley and his longtime partner, Dr. Bartlett, gained certain notoriety in Denver medical circles because they allowed mothers to breastfeed the baby on the delivery table when delivery rooms were the norm. A staff nurse told us this story:

> One of the obstetricians was having trouble with a mother who had just given birth and was bleeding heavily (sometimes happens—even in Natural Childbirth). He told the nurse to get another doctor *fast*. Dr. Bradley happened to be in the hall. He rushed in when called and quickly recognized what was happening. He calmly walked over to where the baby was in a newborn bassinet, picked her up, and put her to the mother's breast for nursing. Then he began to help the

doctor who was using all his medical skills to stop the bleeding. The bleeding was soon controlled by the sucking, undoubtedly, more than the medical skill. The episode made a believer of one more obstetrician.

According to Karen Pryor in *Nursing Your Baby*:

This immediate feeding is deeply rewarding to the mother, as well as being physically beneficial. The firm contraction of the uterus which results, suggests that her intense emotional response to this immediate feeding sets into operation a very strong let-down reflex. The weak and unreliable let-down reflex so typical of many new nursing mothers in the United States may be at least in part a result of delaying the first feeding beyond the critical period.

So, the immediate contractions of the uterus are helping the mother by pulling her uterus back to its normal size and by establishing a good let-down reflex, without which a successful breastfeeding routine cannot easily be established. The let-down reflex allows milk to flow out of the milk glands.

You may frequently hear, "But there's no milk at first anyway," or, "The milk comes in on the third day." Fluid called colostrum is present in the breasts even before the baby's birth. It is a highly nutritious, creamy liquid, low in fat and carbohydrate content, easily digested, and it is known to be rich in immunity factors. It has a cleansing effect on the lower digestive tract. Colostrum will be present in the milk for up to ten days. You want your baby to have this.

It has always amazed me how anyone knows when her milk "comes in." The only way to find out is to take a sample in a clear container and look at it—and how does a mother know what human milk looks like? As a matter of fact, it looks very blue and not like "good, rich" milk at all! So appearance is an unreliable yardstick.

Sometimes your breasts become overfull. Just in case you had triplets, nature is making sure you have enough milk. Or you may become swollen or sore as the milk glands "go into production." They gather all the bodily resources and overdo to the point of discomfort. This lasts only a short time.

Your baby will train your breasts. As his routine settles in, trust your breasts to determine what production is necessary. The milk glands will calm down and produce the right amount of milk for your baby. If the baby is swallowing as he sucks; is having multiple wet diapers a day—then, whether you have milk or colostrum, does it matter? "When the milk comes in" is a cliché often used but it has little impact on mother or baby as it happens. Don't worry! Just put that newborn baby to your breast every time there is a lot of mouthing action and some mewing, whimpering and crying. Do make sure the baby is wide awake and really hungry so that the sucking will be effective.

Looking back over five breastfeeding experiences, I am amazed to realize what we saved. I saved time by not making formula and sterilizing bottles. We saved money not buying milk or formula. I saved myself for each baby. Instead of "propping" a bottle or letting an older child give the feeding, I sat comfortably rocking my baby with no guilt about things not done, because the baby came first.

It's not uncommon for some fathers to feel "left out" from the *breastfeeding couple*. There are plenty of opportunities for the father and baby to bond outside of the feeding times. Be creative—I've always loved it when my little one would gladly fall asleep on her daddy's chest.

The only big disadvantage of breastfeeding is the undeniably self-righteous attitude that we tend to assume. Sometimes it will even tend toward fanaticism. I have always made a supreme effort to hide or cover my feelings, but it is not easy, nor is it always successful. This undoubtedly explains the defensive attitude of some bottle-feeding mothers toward the "Society of Breastfeeders."

Sometimes Breastfeeding Isn't a Fit

All women have the right to bottle feed their baby just as I have the right to breastfeed mine. There must be some innate emotional need to put the baby to breast! Once you hold your baby to breast you really know if it is what you want to do.

Many excuses are given as reasons to not breastfeed and include:

+ There's not enough milk.

+ Some mothers really struggle to get started and may give up too easily. The system is faultless if you are supported as you will be by mothers helping mothers whom you'll find with La Leche League.

+ The baby's sucking will also be a reason often given.

+ Some mothers feel that time is an issue.

+ If the mother is working away from home, she may have the need to let another person take care of the baby.

Even though I can counsel women with problems in breastfeeding, it is important to first establish whether or not she has a true desire to succeed. Without that, sympathizing is the only help they want. I am very good at that, too!

Getting Away

We all feel the need to get away from the baby. Getting away from the children is a legitimate need for mothers. At least once a week, my husband treated me to a night out. During the day, I planned outings with friends. Once breastfeeding is established, it is simple to take the baby with you, but sometimes you need a rest from each other. Give yourself a break when you feel this way.

For an evening out, I would nurse before going and leave a bottle of apple juice or my own expressed milk to be given during my absence. Usually the babies resisted anything so insulting! If they were hungry enough, however, they would take what was offered. It did not seem to hurt them—and I know that I needed that evening out with Richard. The hardest thing to do once you are parents is to have a conversation at home. Too many interruptions!

A trip away from home, if it is for pleasure, is worth putting off until the baby is no longer nursing. We solved the problem once by taking eight-year-old Joe along with eight-month-old Ritchie and had a wonderful time in Montreal, Canada. We left the three girls with my parents. It is always a good experience to be able to spend extra time with one or two children. Joe was a big help with the baby, too. We took turns carrying him in a backpack and we got a lot of attention.

Hard as we breastfeeding mothers try … humility keeps being pushed aside by pride.

One thing all mothers who have breastfed agree upon is that they become better mothers. It will not turn you into the perfect mother, and maybe you will not even become as good as the woman across the street that prefers the bottle routine, but there is an emotional involvement with your baby that is quite wonderful. I have many times had to nurse a crying baby when it did not suit me to do so. I had other things planned for that half hour. Once I sat quietly for a few minutes with baby at breast, however, I would forget all those things I thought needed doing. It can be very nearly a meditative experience!

I remember being furiously, dramatically angry at someone (who and why I can't recall) as I began feeding Allison once. It was therapy for me because my great rage slipped away as I put her to breast. Allison did not seem to have indigestion from it either!

No matter what reason is given, it is my belief that the non-breast fed baby is getting second best.

Bust Booster Exercise

The Bust Booster is one of my "lifetime" exercises. To be used during pregnancy, post-pregnancy and for when the kids are long gone, it will:

1. Strengthen pectoral or chest muscles that help support the breasts.

2. Help to maintain good shoulder posture.

3. Help when you have heartburn and indigestion.

4. Increase blood flow to the breasts; therefore it may be used to increase milk supply.

The pectoral muscles are located beneath and help give support to the breasts. Since the breasts become heavier and bigger with pregnancy and breastfeeding, stronger pectorals are indicated.

Breast tissue is mostly fat deposits surrounding the milk-producing glands and covered by skin. There is no muscle in the breast. This means that breast size cannot be increased by exercise. It also means that breast tissue which sags and stretches cannot be rebuilt—since only muscle tissue can be rebuilt. It is necessary, therefore, to prevent sagging and stretching of breast tissue by good support in a bra. If you prefer to go bra-less, I suggest that you develop a good philosophy about sagging breasts!

The extra weight of your breasts, plus the cuddling position which is frequently used for breastfeeding, tends to pull your shoulders down. The Bust Booster exercise will help strengthen your chest and shoulders to maintain better posture and at the same time relax these overworked muscles.

HOW:

1. Sit in a tailor position on the floor. Support each breast with the inside of each bent elbow.

2. Press your arms against your body as you raise your hands above your head. This gently massages your breasts, stimulating circulation.

3. Lower your arms until your hands are below your waist, slightly behind you, with palms up.

4. Now swing the backs of your hands toward each other, behind you, five times (thumbs up).

5. Bring your hands to your lap.

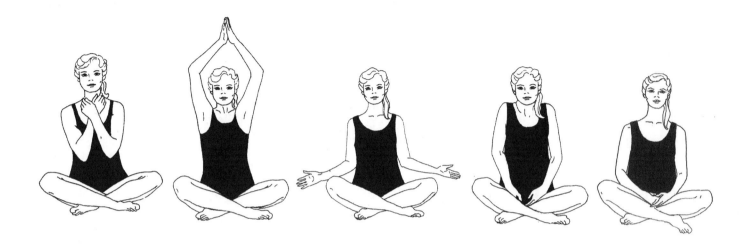

6. Take a deep breath while trying to touch your shoulders to your ears.

7. Let the breath out and the shoulders drop at the same time, while keeping the breastbone high.
   It leaves you feeling very good, somewhat invigorated, and with a relaxed upper back.

WHERE:

Do Bust Booster in private, sitting on the floor, and always in a tailor position so that your chest muscles do the work instead of your back. There are times when steps 6 and 7 can be done to relax your shoulders and upper back without going through the whole exercise. You may need a good stretch in church or in the classroom and this can be done rather unobtrusively. Doing the complete exercise in front of others is sure to create a sensation, however.

WHEN:

During Pregnancy—Do the bust booster approximately three times a day as a chest muscle exercise and to improve your posture. Do it to relax the upper part of your body. It can also be an effective exercise whenever heartburn distress occurs

After the Birth—Use this for increasing your supply of breast milk, wait and see if you need to do it. Try to maintain the three times daily to keep muscles in good tone, but if this brings milk rushing out and creates a problem, avoid using it until you are not oversupplied with milk. If you have a need to create a better milk supply, that is, if the baby seems to demand more milk, then try this to hurry up the process. You will find that it is definitely a help!

Nipple Care:

Nothing can be more discouraging to a new mother of a breast-feeding infant than sore nipples. This condition can be helped by some easy preparation during the last three to four months of pregnancy.

Babies have been categorized according to their sucking, as:

- *Barracudas*—Ouch!

- *Procrastinators*—Sleep for the better part of the first week.

- *Gourmets*—Taste, then smack their lips and taste again before sucking.

- *Resters*—Nurse a bit, rest a bit is their way.

- *Mouthers*—Do lots of testing without much action.

Any group of nursing mothers could make up its own list of "Games Babies Play." There is the "social nurser," who has to take part in whatever is going on in the room while grasping the nipple in his mouth. This is especially common with older babies. There are the "now I have you to myself" nursers. They fuss and won't eat until mom is in a quiet room alone with them.

Because of the "barracudas" especially, you should have nipples that can "take it."

From experience, I've found that soap and alcohol are unnecessary for cleansing and are very drying to the skin. Normal bathing is all you need.

If you live in a dry climate, you need to take extra precautions. Use no soap at all and apply lots of oil to your whole body. Definitely keep soap away from the nipple area.

Preparing Your Nipples

If you do not wear a bra, you will be way ahead on toughening your nipples. From the constant rubbing against clothes, yours will already have lost their tenderness. Topless sunbathing would also be helpful in preparing nipples for breastfeeding. Make sure that you do not have dry and brittle skin. Use a precautionary oil to keep the skin pliable and a sun block is advised.

I would be concerned, for cosmetic reasons only, about sagging breast tissue if you wear no support during pregnancy and breast-feeding. It is not uncommon to have stretch marks along the sides of the breast, because of the increase in size and weight. I personally believe that a good support in a brassiere with a comfortable, wide strap over the shoulder is a good idea. Make sure the bra is big enough in the cup. You may have to get a series of sizes during your pregnancy. Plenty of care in wearing the proper support and lots of lubrication to the skin during breast-feeding and pregnancy should prevent extensive stretch marks and sagging breasts.

Everyone's skin is different and some of you would have no problem with cracking or bleeding nipples even if you made no preparation. Others will need twice as much preparation as I suggest and still be very tender. How the baby sucks will be another factor. A fairly good indication of skin tenderness is how well you suntan. If you tan easily and quickly and never burn, you will probably have very little trouble toughening your skin for the worst barracuda-type nurser. If, however, you burn easily and tan slowly or poorly, it is an indication that much preparation is needed.

HOW:

To have soft, rubbery, pliable nipples use an oily lubricant. You may use vegetable cooking oil, hydrous lanolin, or a cream that you routinely use on your body and know to be good for your skin. Perfumed oils are sometimes irritating to the skin. Lotions containing alcohol are drying. Apply a generous coating all over the breast and on the abdomen, too, to prevent stretch marks. Use your favorite oily lubricant and massage it all around your breasts, nipples, and abdomen then run warm water into the bathtub. Climb in for a relaxing soak. Or, do it during your shower. The warm water will cleanse you (it's amazing how clean and fresh you can stay with no soap—try it!) and rinse off the excess oil from your body while your warmed skin seems to absorb more of the oil. Pat yourself dry with a towel—don't rub—and your skin will feel soft but not greasy. You can dress without a sticky feeling, but it is even more comfortable if the whole routine is done just before bedtime. Do this as often as your skin seems to require the treatment. It should help prevent sore nipples as well as minimize stretch marks on breasts and abdomen.

Rhondda's Tip

Nursing is like the dessert to your pregnancy. It's an extraordinarily special time for you and your baby that reduces daily stress and allows you the time to marvel at the treasure that you have created.

145

Chapter 14

Review, Plan and Practice for the Big Event

Now, when you have at least a month or two until your expected due date, you must use your time wisely with practice sessions. Each night before going to sleep you could "pretend labor" for a few minutes. Together with your coach, do your relaxing. Make sure that your abdominal breathing is as slow and big and loose as possible. Let your coach check you for one-and-one-half-minute practice sessions.

Make sure your position is perfect in every detail. Have your coach run through his relaxation routine so that he becomes sure of himself and doesn't feel self-conscious with the words that make you feel loose and relaxed. Talk it over, and then try again. If you will practice every night from now till labor begins, you will be a good team, ready to handle what your baby has in store for you.

After you've done three or four "relaxing contractions," move on to "pushing" practice. Again, get yourself into position. The easiest way to assume a forty-five-degree squat is with your coach's help.

Coach: kneel on the floor or bed, sitting on your heels. Now your wife can sit at your knees with her back leaning against you. You provide a contour backrest for her.

Next, practice breath holding. Take a first breath and blow it out—take a second breath and blow it out again—take a third breath, pull your legs back and toward your shoulders—put chin on chest and hold your breath as long as comfortable—lift chin—let your breath out fully—take another deep breath, chin on chest, and hold—let your breath out and relax. While you are "pushing," your husband is verbally coaching:

"Keep chin on chest; hold your breath; push down hard; you're doing fine, the baby is coming;
keep up the good work; the pressure is working; you are opening for the baby to be born; etc., etc."

A good length of time to practice for a pushing contraction is one and one-half to two minutes. That is quite long and will make the actual labor rather easy.

> **Warning:** Do not push, since that could contribute to hemorrhoids. Your pushing muscles are strong enough from your lifetime use anyway. The same muscles are used to expel a baby as to expel the contents of the bowel. During practice, then, hold your breath, but don't push!

I've indicated these practice sessions in the order you'll experience them in real labor. But if you're going to get to sleep after this practicing, you might be advised to reverse their order and relax after pushing; then you'll be all ready for a good night sleep. Of course your "coach" deserves a practice session of relaxing and backrub, too, after his work coaching you.

You'll teach each other what is the best relaxing routine by practicing on each other. You must do your bedtime pelvic rocks anyway, so here's a possible routine:

+ Practice pushing together.
+ Practice husband-coached relaxing.
+ Wife relaxes the coach.

- Wife does pelvic rocking as husband crawls into bed.
- Wife gets into bed and both fall asleep.

You will have to decide who turns out the light and when! With all this practice, you will be a super team … you'll be ready for your "Olympics" ahead.

What You Need for the Hospital or Birthing Center

You need to be ready for your trip to the hospital. Pack a small suitcase with your essential needs: gown, robe, slippers, toothbrush and toothpaste, and hair-grooming needs. If you like, you can come home in a gown and robe, but if you want to dress, you may want to take a non-maternity outfit with you—not too tight-fitting, though, as it will take a week or two to get into your usual clothes, maybe longer. For the baby you'll need a warm blanket, undershirt, nightgown, diapers. You probably have a brand new outfit from Grandma, so you may use that if you want.

Now you have your bag packed and under your bed, ready for that exciting day when labor begins!

The Birthing Site

How long you'll remain in the hospital depends on you, your doctor, your hospital, your insurance and who will be at home to help with ordinary housekeeping. The minimum hospital stay in my day was two hours after the baby was born. Non-natural childbirth deliveries were three days and C-sections five. That has changed—most mothers today find that two days is max.

In two hours time mother and baby can be checked by obstetrician and pediatrician and if everything is well you may be discharged to your own bed at home for the best sleep ever, with baby safe and secure in your arms or in the cradle or bassinet beside your bed.

You may prefer a rest in the hospital with nurses to help you take care of your baby and your meals brought to you on a tray. You can keep your baby with you constantly while you have an experienced nurse to call if you need help.

Today, mother and baby usually stay overnight and go home within 24 hours. Since hospitals charge by the day, you have paid for one day anyway! Your hospital stay will be designed by your health care provider, the hospital and you. If you plan to have a home birth then you will have no decisions to make about when to go home! You are staying put! You will have a midwife, probably, and all the necessary arrangements and supplies will be in place. You will be checked on and monitored as is needed.

If you are planning to be at a birthing center, you will most likely leave within eight hours—they are considered outpatient facilities, monitoring both the mother and new baby's well-being until they depart. Usually a midwife is in attendance and will provide postpartum care instructions.

In my day, I remained in the hospital for three days after Joe's birth, my firstborn. I did not enjoy it at all. The hospital care was great, the food delicious and the nurses superior, but I did not like being a patient. Maybe it was because I was a nurse. Also it was not easy to sleep in a strange bed with light and noise down the hall. Remember— you need rest. It was in the days of delivery rooms and nurseries so you can be glad that has changed.

Remember . . . this is your choice. Determine which option is best for you. Plan it and be informed about the details and decisions that must be made.

My baby would be brought to me when he was not hungry and so I had to learn to breastfeed with a sleepy baby. The routine of the hospital did not fit my individual needs. I'd never been in a hospital before as a patient, and, as a nurse, I began to see "hospital rules" in a new light.

By the time Claryss Nan was born, Dr. Bradley had established a new rule. If all was well, we could go home after two hours. Perfect—that was the length of hospital stay that suited me!

If you plan to do the same, I must warn you of a few things. You come home early to rest and have your baby where he belongs—in the family. That does not include all the neighbors' children and their pets—at least not for a week or so.

Your responsibility is to mother your baby so begin now to plan for someone to be there to mother you, the mother.

It's Almost Time!

At seven months, your baby is a real live being now with every part intact and would live if born. He would be very scrawny and thin, five to five and one-half pounds and 15 inches long. The last two months are important to his growth and development. At full term, you would expect him to weigh between six to nine pounds and be about 20 inches long and very, very active. You know just how active he is … it's only a warning bell of what's to come when he emerges!

Your lives are geared to the birth of the baby. All projects are either cleared up before or put off until after the due date. It's actually a super time for getting things done. Being a deadline, it requires organization.

These last few weeks can seem interminable if you just stop everything and wait. With a first pregnancy, keep your life moderately busy and exciting so that the time moves along quickly and easily. Do not overcrowd it, creating a haggard, tired mother for labor!

Some sage words from millions of mothers who've journeyed down your path:

- Try to lie down for a rest at least once a day.

- If you have a toddler during this pregnancy then do the best you can to get extra rest.

- Use the Leg elevation position more often now. Varicose veins could be a problem, so get your legs up as much as ten minutes every hour for painful, aching legs.

- It's O.K. to feel very pregnant and to act it!

- You may be uncomfortable squatting, so do it only when you have to reach to the floor for some reason. That's why you worked so hard to do it well and often earlier in your pregnancy. Now you can do it less often.

- Lifting and bending may cause a contraction of the uterus—so don't feel guilty about asking someone to help you with things. Your husband won't mind lifting your toddler and your toddler can bend over to "pick things up for Mommy."

- Just remember you are already carrying at least twenty extra pounds around with you constantly and you won't be ashamed if you are not anxious to do much extra!

+ Your Pelvic Rock and Tailor Sit will make life far more comfortable. Do your Abdominal Breathing and Relaxing extra times during the day—it's a good rest as well as practice.

+ Your sex life in these last weeks of pregnancy deserves a word or two. Most doctors now agree that there is no great risk of infection from so normal a part of your life. You may find that your lovemaking creates contractions of the uterus. This is perfectly normal and only indicates the sensitivity of muscles getting ready for labor.

+ Pelvic Rocking both before and after lovemaking will aid your comfort. You might be just too big, have too much pressure, and the baby feels too low for you to be interested in intercourse. Husbands will be understanding, and realize that you still need to feel loved, cuddled, and told how wonderful you are. You will desperately need that reassurance! It's not easy to feel confident when your body is absolutely out of control!

Remember, every pregnancy is different! Some of you will feel beautiful, graceful, sexy, and your love life will be fantastic. Perhaps the next pregnancy—same couple—will be the opposite. It can be a warm, fulfilling, happy, loving time in your lives, in spite of any limitations in your sex life, if you'll be understanding of the needs of one another. You'll have a stronger, better relationship from this shared experience. You'll learn a lot more about each other and yourselves. Be loving. Be kind. Be supportive. Be you.

Going Home

Whether you come home in two hours or two days, you should have some help. You need to plan for some help in the home for a while. What type of help will you have? A grandmother to coddle you and the baby would be wonderful, or you could hire some helper to come in for a few hours each morning and tidy up the house, do the laundry and organize the meals. Pay a young girl in the neighborhood to visit after school and play with your toddler for an hour while you and the new baby have a relaxing bath and change clothes to be fresh for the remainder of the day. Help a friend with a new baby with simple housekeeping and preparation of some meals and arrange that she will repay you by doing it for you when your baby arrives. Start planning!

Who will prepare meals? Soup and a sandwich will be a banquet if you feel rested and the baby is not practicing her lung exercises through dinner. Perhaps your husband doesn't mind bringing home take-out dinners for a few days. Your friends may bring you meals as a new baby gift. Start making that your gift to other new mothers now and start the idea going. When my five came along, it wasn't uncommon to see a friend at my door with a big turkey dinner and all the trimmings as soon as we came home with a new baby. A hot meal and all the wonderful leftovers that the family could graze on for days was a perfect gift!

You need some time to enjoy and get used to being a new mother before you return to your role of manager of a household. You are not sick, but you are a new mother with a baby in your arms. You need care and attention and help for a while.

I am making the assumption that if you are a working Mom, you have decent and adequate maternity leave coverage. Maybe you don't. A new baby's needs make for a hectic schedule. Just because you have time off from your job does not mean you do not need extra help in the home. Be smart here—the more help you can get in the beginning, the quicker you will regain your vigor and energy. Meals and cleaning house do not fit in with baby care. I guarantee that your baby's needs and wants are out of sync with the "old normal" routines of your household. Get help.

Rhondda's Tip

Think of this two month time as a form of a dress rehearsal. Plan and organize so that all the extras are finished and ready for you to enjoy the rewards of motherhood. Get organized and plan ahead. For you. For your husband. Enjoy the grand entrance of your baby.

Chapter 15

Let's Talk About the First Stage of Labor

You are now in the final phase of your pregnancy that begins with your seventh month, 30 weeks plus. Your baby is kicking vigorously and lets you know she's quite real. Weighing in at about four pounds, she is looking very much like a newborn baby. Until now, she has been able to turn somersaults in the uterus but with her increased size, there is less freedom. You may feel one spot on your ribs that is being kicked repeatedly and often.

Your baby is becoming more and more a part of your life as a separate personality. She awakens you in the middle of the night because she needs to stretch. You may want to lean into your husband's back and let his baby kick on him for a while so they can get to know each other, too.

If you haven't selected a name, it now becomes more of a need. There is usually a very urgent need by the hospital to register your baby with a real name. "Baby Girl" does not satisfy the hospital lady who has to fill in the form! There are a variety of baby books that can help with your selection—in fact, they become great light, middle-of-the-night reading. Sleeping for a whole night without being wakened by the baby's movements is quite a luxury for any mother-to-be in the post seventh month timeframe.

There are days when you can't wait the remaining weeks until your baby's arrival. She will surely be easier to handle "out" than "in," you decide. There are other days when you wonder if you can possibly be ready for the baby in time. There is uncertainty about your ability to birth and mother this new wee being.

The dad-to-be settles into his role with more reality by now. He usually has become aware of your needs better than you know them yourself. It is such a pleasure for me to be with couples as they anticipate and prepare for this beautiful event in which they will both take part. It is the ultimate intimacy!

Now, too, the realization dawns that it will be up to you, the mother, to allow this increasingly large being to come into the world from the shelter of your body. This acceptance is part of pregnancy and does not seem to occur to you any earlier than necessary. By now you are ready to think about the next stage—it's time to start discussing the actuality of labor.

How Labor Feels

What does labor really feel like? How I wish there was an easy answer to the question. There are as many answers as there are babies. The old smug reply, "You'll know when you are in labor" is not at all true. It was harder to know with our fifth baby than with the first. Experience is not always a help! There are some generalizations and guidelines, however, which will enable you to be pretty sure.

Especially now, we need help from all our friends with experience in childbirth. Listen to all the stories of births that others are willing to tell you. Just remember that yours will be different! Since no two labors are ever the same, it is difficult to tell you how labor feels.

As you hear stories of births from every mother that you know or meet ... everyone loves to tell you their birth story (I also want to share with you my five birth experiences and you will find them at the end of this book!)

There is a strange phenomenon in our culture that women love to suffer in childbirth—as though they *should* suffer! Some of the stories are awful! Almost as if, "I can top you with all the pain and suffering that I had to go through ..." This will make you wish to spend more time with those of us who have had a natural and beautiful experience giving birth.

After hearing some of these horrible, awful stories of births, you will be amazed at the ease of early labor. Relaxed, prepared and knowledgeable women will find that the contractions at the beginning of labor are light and easy and that you are completely comfortable. The tales of pain and horror that you have heard make you expect something very different.

Usually, but not always, labor begins with slow, light contractions, a tensing of the uterus that holds for thirty seconds or less. It may cause you to stop moving because you feel as though you have a heavy weight in your abdomen, but no other sensation. The uterus is very hard and firm and pushed out in front more than usual. When it relaxes, you will go on with what you were doing.

Only after several repetitions of this, within a short space of time, will you realize that it could be the beginning of labor. Now you begin the record of this birth. Write down the time of the beginning of one contraction to the end. Continue to keep a record and you will know how long each contraction lasts and how much time between contractions. This will be the information you will need when you talk to your health care provider. The duration may be thirty to forty-five seconds, maybe even a minute, or more. The time between contractions will be a significant determination of how the labor is progressing.

You may feel a cramping sensation in the abdomen. Sometimes it begins at the top of the pelvis and moves down. Sometimes it begins in the back and moves around into the abdomen. We've had laboring women who mistook their contractions for a stomachache or called the doctor to ask what to do about flu! Anyone who has experienced difficult menstrual cramps thinks beginning labor is too easy to be the real thing. Some women experience labor in their back only. They get a recurring low backache that lasts a short time, then is gone, then comes again, etc. Sometimes absolutely no sensation is felt until it's time to push. That is more the exception than the rule and could be quite a problem when you think about it—no warning that you are in labor! So you see, there are many variations of how labor contractions *feel!*

In other words, don't expect your labor to be "text book." There will be a variety of signs when the "real" thing decides to make its entrance, followed shortly by the star—your baby.

> You know the birth that you want.
>   Expect to have the birth that you want.
>   The alarm is about to go off!
>   Let's get ready to birth this baby!

Signs of Labor

Actual labor shows up in a variety of ways. Physical signs include:
- Beginning of contractions
- The bag of water breaks
- "Bloody show"

Then there are also environmental signs of labor ...

My favorite is the "nesting instinct." Oh so elusive! It is similar to the instinct that animals have to build a nest for the birth of their young or for laying eggs! This is so hard to detect in ourselves because it is a burst of extra energy, something you have not felt for a while and it feels so good! If you have an urge to do a total spring housecleaning and it is November! If it is very near your due date—don't go overboard! It may be that your body is demonstrating a surge of energy which is meant to be available for labor. Saving this energy gets you out of lots of housecleaning, too! If the desire to clean and toss persists, consider hiring a cleaning service to come in and really do a thorough cleaning before your baby comes and save your energy for the hard work of labor which is coming soon.

Beginning of Contractions

When you feel your contractions have started, check in with your health care provider. By now you will have been given some instructions about how many minutes between contractions is the "rule" for you to come to the hospital or birth center. For example, come to the hospital when the contractions are ten minutes apart or less. I once woke up in the night with contractions five minutes apart, so we got ready to go directly to the hospital. I was earlier than I needed to be, but the good news was that I was actually in early labor and not false labor. Sometimes you will be sent home to wait for labor to develop more definitely. It is much easier to do the early part of labor at home where you are at ease and comfortable.

For planning purposes, these are questions you should consider:

+ How far from the hospital do you live?

+ Should you phone ahead to either the doctor or the hospital?

+ What was your past labor experience like, if any?

+ What kind of weather is likely?

+ How reliable is your transportation?

+ What will you do with the other children, if any?

+ What could you do as an alternate plan—if Grandma has the flu, who else could take care of your other children?

+ If your labor begins during working hours, who will drive you?

+ Will your husband come home or meet you at the hospital?

+ Who else could drive you to the hospital?

+ Have you discussed it thoroughly with each helper?

+ Have you found the best route to the hospital/birth center and given it a trial run?

+ If you will be having a Home Birth, how long will it take the Midwife to get to you?

Consider all possible questions now. They are all factors that will seriously affect your peace of mind and therefore your ability to deal with labor. Settle them at once! Plan for all contingencies and arrange suitable alternative plans, then you'll feel comfortable about your approaching due date.

When your contractions become regular or rhythmical, and the time between contractions gets shorter and shorter, it's time for you to head to the hospital—use your own health care provider's instructions. Even when instructions were followed, babies have been born in cars—not always the most delightful or comfortable experience and rather hard on the upholstery! However, it certainly would be a Natural Childbirth!

Big What If ...?

If you live in an out-of-the-way region and are concerned about not making it to the hospital in time, I suggest two things: First, have a serious, frank discussion with your doctor and let him help you solve your problem. Second, a home birth may be the most viable option—your husband or partner will become a key, if not the key member of the birthing team.

If you deliver at home accidentally ... or a venue that isn't the preferred choice ... and an ambulance or other transportation is called to take you and your baby to the hospital, expect to be treated differently than if you had delivered at the hospital. Why? Because an outside delivery is considered "dirty or unsterile"—meaning that there weren't any precautions taken prior to the birth that the hospital would have routinely done as you were admitted.

If a home birth is your choice you will need to find the best midwife in the area who will come to your home for the birth. It will be your responsibility as well as your choice to know what you are doing and be prepared. Also, if there is a chance of a home birth, there are two books that I would recommend that you devour now. The first is Dr. Gregory White's *Emergency Childbirth*. Written in an easily understood manner for the "just in case" time if it should happen that you will be alone for this birth. The second is *Ina May's Guide to Childbirth* by Ina May Gaskin—a mid-wife with over 30 years of experience in home births. Read to acquaint yourself with the natural birth procedures. If you've done neither of these things and you find yourself with an accidental home birth... here are some easy rules to remember:

Call for assistance, then:

+ Do not cut anything.

+ Put the baby to breast with skin-to-skin contact between mother and baby.

+ Keep the baby, mother, placenta and cord together and wait for help to arrive.

+ Bundle up warmly and be sure to contact your doctor!

+ Do not do anything about the placenta and the cord.

Remember … this is your choice, determine which option is best for you. Plan it and be informed about the details and decisions that must be made.

As long as the baby is at breast, nature's method is at work. Unless you are prepared and knowledgeable about a home birth, you will welcome professional help and reassurance as soon as possible.

It will be better if you can manage to get to the hospital or birth center on time and enjoy the security that it affords. You can concentrate on your relaxing and abdominal breathing where you have the safety net in place as planned.

If you are having a home birth intentionally, I would not think any of this would be necessary. You will be well prepared for the birth by your midwife. In the event that she did not get to you before the baby's birth, I am sure she would have given specific instructions so that you would be prepared. I am sure you would call her to come as soon as possible, never the less! The two references above I would suggest you read as preparation, anyway! This is your birth and your responsibility to be thoughtful and prepared for the possibilities you could expect. The "what ifs" should be part of your Birth Plan.

Reminder—if you deliver in an emergency—don't cut anything! Call for help. Wrap the baby and the umbilical cord close to your chest for warmth until help arrives.

Breaking of the Bag of Water or the Amniotic Sac

The baby is floating in salt water enclosed in a membranous balloon called the amniotic sac. The amount of this colorless liquid varies, as does the toughness of the membrane. This accounts for the spontaneous rupture of membranes sometimes prematurely, sometimes during labor and sometimes not breaking at all. Some babies are born with sac, fluid and all intact. In the latter case, the sac must be broken so that the baby can begin to breathe. Superstition claims that a baby born in a caul, as it is called, is truly gifted and will live an outstanding life. Abraham Lincoln, for one, is supposed to have been born in a *caul*—the membrane sac was intact.

So the membrane has to break sometime. It may break early in labor—even before the onset of contractions. It may break during labor. Or the doctor may break it as your labor progresses in the hopes of speeding up contractions.

Sometimes the membrane breaks several weeks early, in which case the doctor will talk to you about inducing labor—that is, use medical means to cause your uterus to contract and start your labor. Your health care provider may have a protocol that is followed when the membranes break early. Make sure you know what it is soon so that you can decide if you like the procedure and will agree with it! You may have to do some research to find out your options and be prepared to present it to the doctor. It usually involves inducing labor with Pitocin after a predetermined number of hours because of a fear of infection. Inductions are rarely pleasant so getting information is important. This protocol is probably put in place due to the hospital's fear of litigation as well as a risk to you and the baby. The maturity of the baby and any signs of early labor will be taken into account. Discuss this with your doctor soon. Make sure you are willing to accept the medical protocol that is required.

How Does It Feel When the Bag of Water Breaks?

There is no sensation other than warm fluid between your legs. Tightening hard on your Kegel muscle helps control it somewhat but not completely. The liquid should be colorless and varies in amount. It did not stain the upholstery when mine broke! You may spill only a cup or so—or you could have gallons—well, it seems like that much! Actually it could be as much as 3 pints. Ordinarily, as long as you are standing or walking, the baby's head will act as a cork pushed into a bottle. The resulting flow will be more like dribbles escaping. If you are lying in bed as your bag of water breaks, you have a much better likelihood of a flood.

We all worry about inundating the supermarket or filling a church pew with amniotic fluid! Usually, the amount is too small to affect others. If anyone around you does realize what has happened, the reaction is always one of wanting to help. You will probably have a dozen offers to drive you to the hospital or you and your groceries home. Childbirth is exciting to us all. Even strangers will want to help.

Once the membrane breaks, you'll probably have to use a towel to sit on, and if appropriate, hold between your legs to absorb the fluid. As you move about there could be more leaking. Other than the leaking there is nothing uncomfortable about it. It does make you excited of course. The baby is coming!

Contact your doctor according to his instructions. Generally, labor will begin within a few hours, if it has not already begun. When the membrane ruptures, the labor usually proceeds more quickly and the baby will be born before too long.

"Bloody Show"

Sometimes you will see bloody show early in labor, or even before you know that labor has begun. In this case, it is an indication that you are dilating and the mucus that has plugged the cervix—the opening end of the uterus—forming a seal, is beginning to come away as the cervix begins to open. This is always present in hard labor and all medically trained persons are familiar with it. Sometimes it is just a heavy, egg-white like vaginal discharge, but it may become streaked or tinged with blood and may even look very bloody to you. This, then, is "bloody show." Here again, check with your own doctor for his rules.

If there is as much blood as a normal menstrual flow, then hurry to the hospital. Bleeding is <u>not</u> normal in labor and indicates a serious problem which must be dealt with immediately.

"Show" is perfectly normal and can be taken casually. Your problem is to know the difference. I suggest that if you are at all unsure, get to the hospital, where help is available. Take no chances!

False Labor

"False labor" is rare with first babies, though certainly possible, and rather common for all subsequent labors. It is a series of uterine contractions which do not continue on to the birth of the baby. Think of it as a practice session for the uterus. There are contractions all through your pregnancy, though you may not be aware of them. They become noticeable as you get closer to your due date. Usually they are sporadic and come one or two at a time. You may be able to cause a contraction by reaching to your top cupboard shelf or by lifting your two-year-old.

These contractions are usually referred to as Braxton Hicks contractions. In false labor, on the other hand, the contractions continue for an extended period at a regular rate. You may cause it by overexertion, or by a particularly stressful day. I would guess that any holiday season gives rise to an increase in false labor.

True labor does not respond or change with your activity. It almost always continues at a regular rate and becomes progressively harder no matter what you do. False labor, on the other hand, will change as your activities change; then will become very irregular, eventually stopping.

What can you do to tell the difference between false and true labor? You do something quite opposite to what you were doing when contractions began. If you wake at night with contractions and you have reason to doubt that it's the real thing, you will suspect it to be false labor. For instance, it may be several weeks before your expected date, or you may have been having lots of activity of the uterus which has not amounted to labor. Get up and move around the house a bit. Time your contractions. Make a cup of tea. A warm calming shower is enough activity to test for true labor. If the contractions continue at a fairly even rate, you are *not* in false labor! If it is false labor, the contractions will slow down and stop and you can go back to bed, well relaxed from your shower.

If you are very busy getting dinner ready for guests, feeding the children, and trying to bed them down before everyone arrives, were up late the night before making preparations and have spent all this day cleaning the house—this is a perfect time for contractions to begin! You must relax and give your uterus a chance to stop being irritated by all your activity. Again, a warm shower would be a good test now. Then lie down for a few minutes. Chances are it is false labor and the contractions will gradually fade out. If they don't, I hope those ten dinner guests are good friends and can have the party by themselves. At least there will be someone to stay with the children!

It can be embarrassing to go to the hospital and have everything stop and have to go home again, but it's a common happening. Doctors generally admit laughingly that most of them have taken their own wives to the hospital in labor, only to be told that it was false. I've yet to hear any statistics on female midwives or doctors about their own labors, but they undoubtedly are not always right either. The point is—don't be embarrassed. It's hard to know if you are in false labor or true. You are the expert on your body and how it feels. Trust your feelings. You can generally determine whether it is time to go to the hospital.

Unless you are happy about the prospect of having your baby at home, if the contractions are regular, getting stronger and more frequent, then calmly go to the hospital or birth center or call the midwife to come to you. Do not worry about false labor!

First Stage of Labor

I have already discussed the early part of First Stage of Labor when I told you how it feels to have labor begin. As the uterus gets a little more eager to empty its contents it increases in intensity.

Do you remember my simple rules for Natural Childbirth?

Rule #1 ... the First Stage of Labor you relax completely and do Abdominal Breathing during the entire contraction. Breathe normally in between contractions.

Rule #2 ... In the Second Stage of Labor you take two deep breaths and exhale each quickly. Take the third big deep breath, hold it, pull your knees up to your shoulders, put your chin on your chest, and keep holding your breath as you bear down to push the baby out. When you can no longer hold your breath, remove your chin from your chest and exhale fully. Immediately take another big breath, chin on chest and hold your breath while pushing as the contraction continues. Repeat as long as you have a contraction. Between contractions breathe normally. You can resume a relaxed position and rest.

Simple, but not necessarily easy!

Now think about being in real labor and imagine that it is becoming harder, more intense and the contractions are coming more quickly and lasting longer. This is a gradual process. At the beginning you will be excited and be talkative and have fun. As the contractions become stronger and more intense you will be more serious and be less chatty. You may feel the need to rest between contractions for the work of the next one. As each contraction begins, you will need to pay attention and consciously relax while diligently paying attention to your abdominal breathing. Remember all the breathing exercises and practices in the beginning chapters? Now you realize how important that was!

Your coach will become more attentive and more aware of your need for his help as the intensity of the contractions progresses. He'll be getting better at helping you to be relaxed—he knows that what he is doing is working for you. His encouraging words and touching improves during your labor and you do better because of his help.

Between contractions, you can tell him what felt best for you. It felt good when he pushed into the small of your back with the flat of his hand which eased your tense back. It felt great when he put a cool cloth on your forehead between contractions. You needed the feather touch on your abdomen to remind you of the breathing. You become a well matched team. You listen to what you are told and it makes it easier than doing it on your own. He can keep you aware of time and that the contraction is about to begin or end. Together you can do this. The contractions get harder and harder but you are at the top of your game, a well-conditioned athlete with a coach who understands your needs.

Let us pause for a bit of explanation about what is happening within your body during this time. The uterus is made up of total muscles. With a contraction, the uterus tightens from the top down toward the cervix which is closed by bands of muscle which circle the opening and are there to keep the uterus closed while you are pregnant. So the work of the uterus is to force the cervix open and it is a fight—the cervix thinks its job is to stay closed; the uterus is saying—your job is done ... move aside, I've got a big job here. The best thing for you to do to help with this process is to relax completely and let the uterus do what it needs to do—get the cervix open to allow for the final birthing. It is usually a slow and gradual process and there are two measurements that let the staff know how fast your body is getting the job done.

This brings up another discussion with your health care provider that needs to be added to your Birth Plan and list of questions. What are the expectations of the frequency of these vaginal exams? There is always a risk of infection when anything is introduced into the birth canal. It is best to keep this procedure to a minimum.

First, There is Dilation or Opening of the Cervix

Your health care provider can check the opening of the cervix with a vaginal exam by using fingers to measure. The measurement is commonly in centimeters from zero to ten. The largest, ten centimeters, is considered the size that will allow the baby's head to push through into the birth canal also called the vagina.

It must be obvious that all these measurements are subject to interpretation of the person whose hand is feeling the cervical dilation. Also the term "fully dilated" must be measured more by the size of the baby's head than by a measurement in centimeters. Full dilation causes your body to begin pushing. It would be unusual for you to miss the very strong urge that this dilation creates in your body. It's an urge that is impossible to resist. Once you start pushing you are in the Second Stage of Labor.

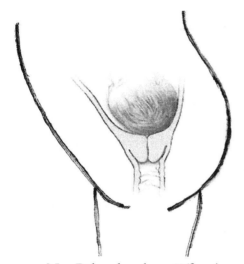

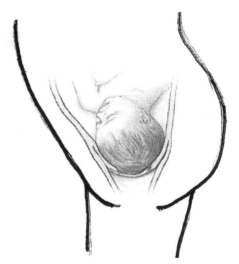

Not Dilated and not Effaced   Dilated and Effaced

Also There is Effacement or Thinning of the Cervix

The other measurement that is used to check your progress in labor is called *Effacement* or *Thinning*. The cervix does not open like the neck of a bottle, but rather like a turtleneck sweater. As the walls of the cervix thin out to become tight over the baby's head, dilation, or the opening of the cervix will happen much faster. Once the cervix has thinned, it will dilate more quickly … sometimes surprisingly quickly!

It can be disappointing to discover that you've worked so hard at relaxing for a long time and you are only dilated to three or four centimeters. But, if you are thin or well-effaced, you could be further along than if you are six centimeters and thick! Once the thinning is complete, the uterus will be very efficient at dilating the cervix and you will be pushing before you know what is happening.

Review and Go Forth ...

Imagine that you are in the beginning of First Stage of Labor. You have been admitted to the hospital and have gone through all the necessary procedures. You and your husband may now walk the corridors of the obstetrics ward or Birth Center while you go through the early stages of dilating. Walking is a gentle way of moving into stronger labor. When a contraction begins, you will bend slightly forward and rest your arms against your husband as you relax and breathe abdominally. Your uterus can fall forward and you will be more comfortable than in an upright standing position. As the dilation and thinning progress and it becomes uncomfortable walking, it is time to return to your room.

You are the one who will decide when it's time to get into bed so that you can relax completely and breathe abdominally with each contraction. Be sure to be in the side-lying relaxation position that you've been practicing. There is often a clock on the wall so your husband can time your contractions and keep your birth record.

It is helpful to get relaxed and loose and begin abdominal breathing 15 to 20 seconds before you expect a contraction. You get a head start! When the contraction is over, you can wiggle and move about or sit up and continue your conversation with your husband. Your activities between contractions will change as your labor progresses. The harder and closer together the contractions are, the less likely you are to need anything to do. You will no longer be playing cards! Remember to move your arms and legs, though, to relieve tension and increase circulation to your extremities.

Your husband will have his real test of love at this time. The more work relaxing is, the more you need him. If he can be very vocal, it is a help. He can whisper relaxing and encouraging things in your ear. If that is hard for him, have him read my poem on relaxing found in this book—*Limp and Loose, Warm and Heavy*—or some other written piece that helps you stay relaxed. One coach had a unique idea for relaxing his wife; he sang ballads to his own guitar accompaniment. Not all of us have husbands with that particular talent, but they are all talented in knowing how they can help relax the woman they love.

Another benefit of Natural Childbirth is getting to know things about each other that nothing else could ever teach you!

Back rubbing is another act of love. Many husbands perform heroic feats of arm strength in this way. One easy and comfortable way to relieve back pressure during labor is to press the palm of his hand against the tailbone area (lower back) where it feels best to you. It's easier on your skin and may feel better than rubbing.

Each night, as you prepare for bed, you should rehearse together. Pretend that you are having a contraction and let your husband practice his skills at relaxing you and seeing that your abdominal breathing is very slow and deep. You may have lots of clowning around and laughter as you learn to do these crazy things together but it will help you get ready to work as a team when you are actually in labor!

Here are the big benefits to all of this when you in labor:

+ You've found out what works and do not have to waste time and effort figuring it out.

+ You can give helpful suggestions when you practice.

+ Your husband can learn to avoid the ticklish spots and can leave out irritating words.

+ You may like his hand on your abdomen as a reminder with your breathing.

+ You may not like his hand on your abdomen with your breathing.

+ You may like a soft touch here and there to help you loosen parts of your body.

+ You may like an idea of how long the contraction has been going.

"It's thirty seconds now, halfway through." Practice together. If he is really a coach, he won't wait until the final game time to begin working with the star player. No athlete wins laurels without a coach, or without working very hard with her coach!

Another aspect of your husband's being a strong coach in labor is that it shows immediately to the hospital staff. They realize that you know what you are doing. You'll probably get lots of cooperation from the staff because they see how well you are working together.

It is Time to Make a Birth Plan and Add to Your List of Questions for the Doctor

Birth plans are often used to help you know what you want in labor. It is also a way to communicate to your Health Care Provider what you expect.

Please, read this chapter again, now, with a pen and paper ready.

+ Make a list of your Questions for the Doctor.

+ Make a list for your Birth Plan.

Now you have a good start on both those 'To Dos'.

Rhondda's Tip

The first stage of labor has so many variables … be ready … it will be a very special experience. Guaranteed, each labor will be different from another—unique in sequencing, time, what you feel and what you experience. Every labor will be a once in a lifetime experience. Appreciate it!

Chapter 16

Transition ... The Wild End of the First Stage of Labor

Now you have come to the end of the first stage of labor which is called transition. You are probably dilated between 7 and 10 centimeters. Transition is that intermediate period when you are almost through first stage and almost into second stage. Your body doesn't have it quite sorted out! There is nothing to do but help the body make the decision. Keep relaxing until you can't do it any longer. You will at some point know that you must push!

Remember, relax completely and breathe abdominally with each contraction in first stage. You've been doing just that until now and you are becoming better at it all the time. It is what will keep you comfortable through transition as well. Transition is the hardest part of labor, but it is also usually the shortest part.

Transition is unpredictable. It was never the same twice in my five births. Because of this I will divide you into three groups according to the way you will probably experience transition:

1. Some of you will never know you went through it. You were dilated to 7 centimeters one minute and your cervix dilated completely with the very next contraction. Your uterus did the work too quickly for you to be aware of it. Suddenly you are ready to push; you really never had a Transition Stage.

2. Some of you will be working so hard at relaxing that you will not be aware of anything but a gradual increase in intensity of your labor. After the baby is born, and you and your husband are reminiscing,

you will be able to recognize where it was that your transition took place You will remember some of the symptoms that I am about to describe to you.

3. Then there is the third group. Everything gets messed up! You need a good understanding of transition so that you don't become discouraged and "give up." You need strong support to maintain your relaxation. Your husband will earn a trophy for coaching you through it. For you, in the third group, here's an explanation of transition:

During transition, the uterus does its most difficult, most violent work. It is contracting very hard and rather quickly. Sometimes contractions will come as close together as one minute and last about as long. Sometimes the intervals will increase in length during this time, however. It can be very confusing. Expect that all you can do is what your uterus dictates.

During pregnancy, your body increases the volume of blood in your body by about one third. The uterus grows, as you are well aware, and needs a full blood supply to take care of the functions it performs supplying a growing fetus with nourishment.

When you have a hard contraction in this stage of labor, the muscles of the uterus squeeze so hard that much of that one third extra blood rushes out into your other blood vessels. This makes you hot and flushed. You may appear to be blushing. You will become uncomfortably warm. Every capillary in your body has extra blood in it and this makes your nerve endings very irritable indeed—so as your husband rubs your back and puts his hand on your tummy to coach your breathing, you feel a distinct desire to hit him. Even the nightgown and bed covers are irritating. All these unpleasant sensations—while you are working so hard at relaxing and breathing abdominally with a very hard contraction! It takes extreme concentration to relax.

Ahhh! Now the contraction is ending and you can take care of these unpleasant circumstances. But wait—things are changing. All that blood racing around in you is needed by the uterus again to get ready for its next contraction. Blood rushes back to fill those large veins and arteries in a momentarily loose uterus. Suddenly you feel rather light-headed and dizzy. Not a bad sensation, but it makes you forget to get ready for the next contraction. Oh, dear, that pizza you ate before you knew you were in labor is getting very restless. Perhaps you'll have to give it up, as your body can't have a baby and digest a meal all at the same time.

If you do throw up, it is inconsequential compared to the other things you are doing just now! Now what? You are trembling. You're not cold but your body is acting as though you are because you are shivering. The obvious solution is to add an extra blanket. Poor labor coach. If you've been able to give verbal commands as fast as things are happening in your body, he'll think you've lost your mind! In a way he would be right! The volume of blood rushing into and out of your brain makes you dizzy and slightly disoriented. Your poor brain first has too much blood and then not enough as the body deals with the needs of the uterus. So you are a bit crazy for that short time!

Please realize that the baby's blood supply is totally independent from all this activity in the mother's body. The baby's blood supply is NOT compromised in any way.

Now you begin another contraction and the whole cycle repeats itself. Well, not quite—you probably will not vomit more than once, if that.

Fortunately, you've practiced very hard at relaxing and your husband is offering encouragement and lots of verbal energy. Before you know it, you may feel as though you need to have a bowel movement. That is an indication that the baby is low enough to be pressing against the rectum and that Second Stage of Labor has begun.

181

Or you may take a nice, big abdominal breath and then not want to let it out. You may even begin grunting. These are all signs of second stage labor.

Signs of Readiness to Push:

You take in a good abdominal breath and then just hold it.

You feel the need to have a bowel movement.

You begin grunting!

You simply can't help pushing.

Looking back over five labors, I developed a composite picture of transition, by far the most unique stage of labor. It was the hardest part, requiring every ounce of energy and control I had. I tried every gimmick I ever read in a book or heard from any teacher I'd met. I always came back to abdominal breathing and total relaxation as the best relief in transition.

Also, I would get very restless and run to the bathroom between contractions to empty my bladder. Of course, I got caught there with a contraction more than once! What you find out as you are on your hands and knees on the bathroom floor with a hard-as-a-rock uterus is that it hurts a lot, but it only lasts about one minute. Then you can get back to bed and be ready for the next contraction. What the human female body can do in the birthing process is truly a miracle! Appreciate it! Appreciate you!

By the way, do NOT run to the bathroom if you have the urge to empty your bowels! That is a sign of being ready to push. You do not want to give birth to your baby into the toilet!

Transition brings on a psychological change, too. I was, all at once, this angelic creature giving birth—a Madonna in touch with Creation. I lay in shining light and was above all others—and why in the "blankety-blank" was my husband not coaching me properly? Who does he think he is to put his head down on his arms to rest at a time like this? Ring for the nurse—get me the doctor—I do not want to be ignored!

I can laugh now, but nothing was funny then. I hope I'm giving you enough warning so that you'll be able to deal with this very short time in your labor. Don't let a few minutes ruin the next wonderful stage. If you are being tempted to accept the drugs being offered to "take the edge off," … *Dont.*

> You are almost there.
> You can see the finish line.
> A few steps more and you will be on the mountain top!

Those drugs will harm your baby. It will make him sleepy and you will lose the alert bonding time with your baby. There are far worse possible results! It is a huge drug overdose for your baby. You have come this far and the pushing is the next step, you are so close to the best part. You have no idea the harm that could come to both of you from the drugs that are being offered.

Before you get to this stage in your labor you <u>must</u> find out about the harm the drugs can cause. Do your research now so you know what problems you might cause to you and your baby with the use of drugs.

If you give up and feel that you need medication you will lose control. You will have to stop all the good work you are doing. You will have to wait for the anesthetist to come. You will have to be put into an uncomfortable position while the procedure is performed. You will have to wait a few minutes for it to take effect. Meanwhile your body continues with good hard contractions but you can't relax with them as you are busy doing as you are told for the procedure to be performed. Then ... nothing!! No feeling whatsoever! No wonderful sense of giving birth to your baby. You will delay your birth by an hour or more as your body stops the natural process of labor. You may get some rest but you still have a baby who needs to be born. You have given up control of your birth.

You will have lots of approval from the medical staff. The staff is always happy to take over and do what they are trained to do. It validates their importance.

Transition is a short time in labor so do not give up now. You and your coach can finish this together.

Add to your Birth Plan that you request the staff not to *offer* any drugs. That could stop some of the harassment. You will ask for them if it is your need. Then together make a plan for giving yourself time to consider whether you really want to be drugged or not. You could agree for instance, that when you feel you'd like help, you will go through eight more contractions. Then reassess the level of difficulty of the contractions. By then you and your coach can make a realistic decision together about how you will proceed with the birth.

Think of your labor as a freight train. Each boxcar or contraction is a separate entity. It is joined securely to the boxcars on either end All are needed to make a train—but some might be empty or even need to be put off on a siding and left behind. It changes the train very little. All your contractions are linked together to form labor. If you mess up one or two, it's not the ruin of your whole labor. You have time between contractions to get yourself together again and be ready for the next one. You get back on track and continue a successful labor. Give yourself a pat on the back for the contractions you handle well and forget the ones you flubbed. No woman alive is going to be perfect with every single contraction in labor.

I know from experience that we berate ourselves for the bad, but please give yourself credit for the good instead!

Pushing Is Such Joy!

Do not give up and miss the best part

Pushing is hard work but it does not feel as hard as transition contractions. In transition, you are just about ready to enjoy pushing. You are moments away from the grand finale. You will feel your baby push his way into the world … into your waiting hands! Experience the great feelings of joy as you push! Be in on the fun of the cheering section as everyone yells at you to Pusssssh! Feel the pressure and then the release.

You are so close! Do not rob yourself of the *Best Part*!!

Do not give up during transition! You can do it! You are ready to push your baby into the world! This is what your body was made to do! Take responsibility for this act! You have prepared for this. You have worked so hard to reach this point in labor. You are right at the peak of the mountain. You have only a very short way to go. You can make it to the summit! Do not rob yourself of the best part of having a baby! With transition, you are nearly at the peak of the mountain.

Rhondda's Tip

You need to become aware of the harmful effects of routine drugs that will be offered to you during labor. Do your homework! Recognize the extreme overdose your baby will get from an effective dose of a pain killing drug for you. Check out the scientific research that has been done. Do not believe that drugs are safe for you or your baby. Your body is made to give birth. The baby who is alert and ready to find your breast will be your reward. Keep that darling baby's wellbeing in mind.

Chapter 17

Pushing into the Second Stage of Labor

Now, let's begin our discussion of second-stage labor. Pushing is work!

Once your labor reaches the end of transition, which is the end of first stage of labor, a major change takes place. It *feels* very different and you act differently.

Second stage means the cervix is fully dilated to allow the presenting part of the baby, usually the head, to come down into the vagina or birth canal. Now the passive first stage is over for you. The second stage is usually shorter than the first stage (note—I did not say always shorter). Second stage is a time for strenuous activity and total involvement with the work going on inside you.

> Rather than trying to keep out of the way of the working uterus, as in the first stage, now you will make your strong pushing coincide with the effort of the uterus. The result is that the second stage will be as efficient as possible.

How do you know when it's time to begin pushing?

I have already given you some guidelines for this in previous chapters.

There can be a variety of reactions that you could experience.

Some of you will be absolutely sure that you are in second stage and will begin pushing despite your coach's great efforts to calm you and keep you relaxed.

No one else knows what you know!
Your body does not allow you to do anything other than hold your breath and push!

Trust me, your coach doesn't know that you are ready to push. Your coach has become so very good at relaxing you by this time that he may be upset when you refuse to do what he (or she) says. He reminds you to relax … but you begin holding your breath and bearing down. If you have no doubt that it's pushing time, go ahead and push, but for heaven's sake, tell the nurse or doctor what you are doing. As Dr. Bradley use to say, "Push the bell first and your bottom second."

Some of you may be much less certain that it's time to push, but you think it is. Try to relax while you get the doctor or nurse to make sure that you are fully dilated. Pushing too early will slow down the process some, as it causes a swelling of the tissue and hardens that lovely soft cervix you worked so hard to create. If in doubt, get a professional opinion. Or wait until you really can't avoid pushing.

There are no "normals" in labor. Have I made that very clear by now?

You may never have a subjective urge to push and will need coaching to know when the uterus is contracting. That is when you need to be pushing!

You may also valiantly carry on with your relaxing even though it is not very effective any longer. It is not a problem to the baby if you continue to try to relax but you may feel that there is nothing to relax about.

At this stage, you may find yourself feeling downright cranky and irritable with those who are trying to make you as comfortable as possible.

The result of all this confusion is that you may believe Natural Childbirth is not for you. This is where the allure of drugs sounds enticing because it hurts **not** to push. When you are pushing actively, all you feel is pushing. If you are feeling as though you have pain, then you are not pushing hard enough.

My advice: Push through the pain! You will have no time or need to ask for anesthesia. *Your baby is nearly here!* Everyone gets very excited when the head becomes visible as you push and you will have a huge spurt of energy. The finish line is truly in sight.

Another possibility is that you may be aware of a change but not an urge to push. This is where the health care provider will be of great help. Those around you can usually sense the change in your breathing. Also your attitude will noticeably change. It is time to check your dilation to verify that you are indeed ready to push.

Your labor coach undoubtedly sensed the change, too, but without experience may not have known what it meant.

A close friend had this experience: Anna mistook the beginning of labor for "gas pains." Her husband was wise enough to bring her to the hospital—just in case, as quite a few hours had gone by. As they were being admitted to the hospital, Anna was sure that she was a "failure" because she was so lousy at relaxing. A few minutes later, the doctor discovered that she was well into second-stage labor—and she thought she was doing badly! Once told to push, she did magnificently and soon gave birth to a baby boy. As the three of them walked out of the delivery room (yes, she walked out), she looked up at her husband and said, "Well, honey, what else shall we do today?"

If You Are a First Time Mother …

At this point, I must talk to the first-time mother separately from the mother who has already given birth to one or more babies. The reason for this is that the first birth will take longer in second stage than subsequent births. The birth canal or vagina is a much less muscular area than the uterus. Therefore, once the birth canal has been pushed open and stretched by a normal-size baby, it will allow a baby to pass through more easily the next time.

Since the uterus is all muscle, it can tighten up to its maximum strength so your second labor *could* have a longer first stage than with the first baby. In most cases, it's usually slightly shorter. Second or third babies may have longer or shorter first-stage labors, but the second stage of labor will likely be shorter than with the first baby. How well you push will make a difference, of course. Other variants could be a tired mother, a large head, the baby's position, and a premature birth, to mention a few. We have more exceptions than rules in baby birthing!

Generalizing, then, if this is your first baby, you'll be left on your own to push until the baby is closer to the opening of the vagina (in other words, farther along in the birth canal). You will be made comfortable but the staff will remain calm. You can have the head of the bed up so that you are in a near sitting position or in an "almost squat" position for pushing. Between contractions you will lean back into the contour shape of the bed and rest.

As a contraction begins, you will take two preparatory breaths and let them out fully. With the third full breath, pull your knees back toward your shoulders, elbows up and out, hold your breath, and with chin to your chest, bear down with all your strength. If it hurts, you probably aren't working hard enough. The hard, steady pushing obliterates all other sensations in your perineum and abdomen. Think strong!

Push as hard and as long as you are able until you can no longer hold your breath. Release your chin from your chest (raise your head, in other words), let your breath out completely, and if you still feel some contraction in the uterus, take another huge breath, chin to chest, pull legs out and back … and keep pushing. You'll *know* if you try to stop pushing too early. That contraction will be very apparent without your pushing pressure. It's almost too amazing to believe until you do it, but it works!

Pushing Is As Pushing Does

About the time your baby's head begins to be visible as you push—"Caput is showing"—the medical professionals who are attending you will now begin to show some excitement and hasty preparation for the imminent arrival of your baby. If your baby has hair, anyone observing the vaginal area will most likely comment on seeing the baby's dark hair!

However, if you are a "multip", a mother with multiple births, when you say you are ready to push, everybody goes wild. Your baby could arrive with only two pushes and it's considered a "failure" of the staff if you should have your baby before they are ready!

Never mind what is going on around you.

Continue with your pushing as I've described several times now!

Push strong, long and hard.

If you are feeling pain, you are probably not pushing hard enough. I know, I know ... I've said this before.

Most hospitals are extremely conscientious about having the baby arrive into a sterile world. The doctors have been trained to deliver babies in a prescribed manner and you will have learned about that on your hospital tour. Any changes that you wanted were discussed with your health care provider and made part of your Birth Plan.

Now is NOT the time to do anything but push hard. You may have a contraction as you are instructed to do something or other. **Do nothing during a pushing contraction except PUSH.** You will be extremely uncomfortable when you do not push with a contraction. The uterus is a big strong muscular organ and when it squeezes on the baby to push it out, you will feel the strength of it ... unless you push with it to help do the job of getting the baby out into the world. It will make you sympathetic to any woman in labor that was not taught to push.

Where Will All This Activity Take Place?

You have become acquainted with how the Birthing room is used during your pushing stage if you toured the facility. These are details that you will discuss with your Health Care Provider early in your pregnancy while at an office visit. Make your wishes known.

The Birthing room bed will be changed to accommodate the birth process. There will be leg holders put in position so that you can rest your legs in them between pushes. During a push, always get into the squat posture, with legs pulled out and back, chin on chest. As soon as the doctor is in his place with you, the end of the bed/table is lowered so that your bottom is at the edge. It is the same as the examining tables in the doctor's office. The doctor will put sterile sheets around you so that he has a sterile (as clean as possible) area for the birth of the baby. Your doctor will explain to you any rules that he finds important and your coach will remind the staff of any agreements that you made with your Birth Plan. What is important now is that you are allowed to push properly to give birth to your baby.

As the doctor is organizing his part of this exciting procedure, your husband-coach is doing his thing by helping you be the best pusher in the whole world. One thing is necessary to be completely ready for pushing. Get the head of the bed raised so that you are almost sitting up. Of course, you don't want to fall off the end of the bed. Work with the staff and coach to get the right position for pushing. I've found that a forty-five degree angle is optimum for pushing. This affords a downhill slide for the baby, allowing gravity to help you with your pushing. You open the birth canal most effectively in this position. It is also easier to push.

You may be able to actually squat for pushing, as in an "on your feet" squat and there will be a procedure in place for you to do that if you agree on it ahead of time. Get your lists ready!!

Remember the Butterfly exercise? You will find that the Butterfly is the perfect exercise to make you ready to be comfortable with the pushing position. Review it and make sure you are practicing. Find a special time at the end of the day and have a little fun with it—these exercises have enormous payback for both you and baby.

Here is a Review!

With each push, begin by taking two breaths and letting each one out. As you take your third breath, which you will hold, pull your knees back and toward your shoulders, elbows up and out. Hold firmly to your legs with your wrists under your knees so you can't slip out of position. Bear down firmly and steadily, with your chin to your chest. Your husband has his arm around your shoulders, helping you keep your back bowed, and is verbally coaching and encouraging you all the time you are holding your breath and pushing.

Once you are in this position, verbal coaching will sound something like this:

"Put your chin down, hold your breath, push hard, relax the Kegel muscle, push hard, that's great, you're doing a good job, keep it up, push hard, keep pushing, make sure you're relaxing that baby door, the baby is coming, we'll soon have a baby, great pushing, you're doing well, keep pushing, *puussshhhh!!*"

He keeps this up at a fast, enthusiastic pace as though he were actually a coach of a foot race, spurring on the contestant. Who could help but do a good job with that kind of encouragement!

I recommend that you practice this out loud with lots of repetition and do it often, now, as you practice and before you need it in labor. It's a great way to get ready for this exciting event. The coach can be a very crucial and important member of the team. Good coaching can make all the difference. The staff will recognize how prepared you are to have this baby naturally and with control—and they will be less likely to interfere or even sabotage the process and your plans for a Natural Childbirth. They will appreciate that you know what you are doing to help your baby be born. How proud you'll be of your teamwork and your baby!

As you are doing this hard, efficient pushing, the doctor is watching your perineum to see how well the skin is stretching. When the skin becomes very shiny, tight and white, it will tear if nothing is done. Perhaps you will be asked to push less hard until the perineum has a chance to stretch. This is another detail to discuss early in pregnancy. The medical judgment may be to do an episiotomy. This is a subject of a great deal of controversy. I recommend you find out all you can about it before you decide how you feel about the issue. Check your Midwife's ideas and look at *BradleyBirth.com* for current guidelines. Do not let this be a surprise. Talk about it and read up on it. Make sure you like the protocols followed by your health care providers before you agree to hire them.

> Your Birth Plan is an important part of getting the birth you want!
> How can it be what you want unless you know what you want!
> Again, I say, go through this book, chapter by chapter, and write on your lists everything that you want and that you need to ask and that you have to investigate for you to have the Best Birth Ever.
> That is your Birth Plan! You have to have expectations to reach your goal!

Your Prince or Princess Is about to Arrive!

The baby's head is now "crowning"—pushing hard against the skin of your perineum and even causing it to bulge. The outer tissues, including the skin, are tough and hard to stretch. This is partly the nature of the skin and partly due to our maintaining a constant covering there. During pregnancy, you can prepare this area by using lots of oil and very little soap. Constant tailor sitting, Kegeling and squatting will increase the elasticity of the perineum, also. There is a natural numbness with the baby's head crowning and with your very hard pushing. If the doctor finds it necessary to do an episiotomy, he will cut during a contraction and while you are pushing. Or it is possible that you will tear. In either case, you will not feel it! There will be a release and probably with that same contraction, the baby's head will be born.

There is no reason for giving any kind of anesthetic for an episiotomy. As long as you are pushing, you do not feel any pain, so why administer a "painkiller"? It's too late to give an anesthetic. Pain would be created by the procedure intended as the remedy. Any anesthetic, even a local, would be absorbed by the baby. In a few seconds, that very powerful adult dose of relaxant would be in your baby when he needs all his energies for beginning life!

If you have an episiotomy or tear, a local anesthetic will be needed to repair you with sutures. The natural numbness created by your hard pushing and the crowning of the head will be gone by then. When the baby is born and the cord is clamped, the local anesthetic will no longer be a threat to the baby and is safe for you.

Sometimes an episiotomy is not needed. The doctor should not automatically cut you, but will make a medical decision in each case.

Remember:

Any questions that deal with the actual birth should of course be added to your Birth Plan and List of Questions for your health care provider. When you attend your Bradley classes, you will get lots of help from the class members as well as the Instructor. Most of your questions will be discussed in class and you will have information to help you make your decisions. There is tremendous advantage to attending the Bradley Method Classes I hope you are able to attend them.

Rhondda's Tip

Nothing in your life, to date, prepares you for the extreme joy of hearing your baby cry and call out to you as he emerges from your body. Then the thrill of holding that precious being as your eyes lock … oh my, it is so exquisite. Let no one rob you of the moment!

Chapter 18

The Birth of Your Amazing Baby

Now you are ready for your baby's head to be born. This is the actual moment of birth for the mother. Your work is done, and a flood of joy, accomplishment and love overwhelms you.

You may be conscious of a very tight stretched feeling in the perineum or specifically at the rectum. Now is the time for decisions about the need for an episiotomy or not. This will be a choice you and your doctor will have discussed in detail as you made your Birth Plan. There are these two options:

- You may continue to push through the contractions and take the risk of a tear in the perineum. Your perineum may stretch easily and comfortably over the baby's head with no damage at all!

- You may expect the doctor to make the decision about whether or not to do an incision to prevent tearing if it is necessary. There is no doubt that this will be the only choice that is totally acceptable to the doctor.

She will want to be in control!

You will not be aware of the incision the doctor makes or a natural tear. You might feel a release of pressure in the area that was so stretched … but that is a relief and not pain.

Have you noticed my differentiation between pain and other sensations of the laboring experience? To me pain is a symptom of something very wrong in your body, whereas *labor* is a normal, natural function of your body. It is a sensation that you understand and can manage.

Do the right things and you are able to be comfortable or at least find it tolerable.

Do the wrong thing and you are in pain!

Sometimes the contraction is over as the head is born so the baby's body is still in the birth canal. This is a strange feeling for the mother and a rather anxious moment for the father, as he doesn't feel he has a baby until he sees the whole body. Now you must wait patiently until the next contraction allows you to push the body of your child into the world.

Some doctors will help you to reach down and lift the baby out of the birth canal yourself as soon as the shoulders have been delivered. The closer you can get to your baby, the better! Or perhaps you have elected to have the father help in that final birthing moment. These are also to be added to your Birth Plan.

With the last push, tension is high in the room. I think there is never a nonchalant nurse, midwife or doctor at the moment of birth. It is always a miracle. So don't be surprised if tears are streaming down all your faces! The sex of your baby will be exciting, too, even if you know what to expect. The room will be filled with lots of emotion; laughter and joy. You will feel pride of accomplishment and there is nothing to compare with the pleasure of holding your baby in your arms for the first time.

The father is proud of his child, himself and especially his wife. If there are friends or family members in the birthing room, they will be beaming as well—almost as if they were major factors in the big production. You, the mother, have become overwhelmingly maternal in an instant. You beam at your husband/partner, smile tenderly at his masculine tears; kiss any part of him you can reach, his hand, his sleeve, his lips when offered! And you reach for your baby and coo and talk baby talk to this funny little bundle.

A Final Task and an Essential Beginning

As soon as you can reach your baby the most important thing you can do is to slide the baby, amniotic fluid, blood and all, up your abdomen, up to your breasts. Let the baby move to whatever part of your breasts or tummy is the preference. Both the father and mother should be rubbing the baby and moving all the slippery fluid about on their hands and arms and body. This has been discovered to be a major contribution to bonding with the baby during this alert time in the newborn's life.

Bonding is forever! It is considered to be the touch and smell that are so important for this bonding experience. This can be taking place while the cord is still in place.

You definitely need to put this in your Birth Plan and may have to find the research to support your request. I am not sure how widespread this idea is! It is enthusiastically supported by the Bradley Method. This will also have to be arranged with the nursing staff.

Meanwhile, the cord is clamped and cut. Many fathers participate in the cutting of the cord as their part of the final birthing.

These first moments of having a baby out of your body and into your arms are unforgettable.

+ Nothing is more important at this time than to have the baby in your arms and at your breast.

+ This is the most active, alert time of this newborn.

+ It will last for at least an hour.

+ Your baby will look searchingly into your eyes and lock into your soul.

+ This is the moment of imprinting.

+ This will define your relationship for life together.

+ Whoever holds your baby in that first hour will be imprinted with your child.

+ Make sure the right people are with you at the moment of birth.

+ Do not let anyone take this precious time away from you and your newborn.

In the hospital environment, the nurses routinely weigh and measure your baby; pretty him up a bit before handing your baby to you. In a birthing center, the mother is usually given the baby immediately after birth. Do not allow any procedure to be more important than allowing your baby to imprint with you. The baby needs to be put in your arms. Make a fuss! Yell and scream! Demand to hold your baby! You must spend a few minutes gazing into your baby's eyes even if the medical staff thinks there is urgency to their procedures. Nothing is more important than you and your baby getting to know one another.

Cleaning up, weighing and measuring can come later. Make sure you add this to your birth plan and inform your doctor ahead of time so the nurses don't scoop him up and away from your waiting arms. Think how confusing this can be to the baby. The important people in his life need to get to know him at this time.

The father can follow the baby if the health care professionals take him away from you in spite of your protest. The father could carry his baby and use this as a time to gaze into each other's eyes and bond to one another. Please be aware of the importance of this first hour with your baby.

> The procedures above will probably not be allowed unless you are completely drug free. If you've been drugged or medicated you will not be considered a safe place for your baby, the baby will not be alert and awake and you will be somewhat impaired and compromised so that you are not able to demand your rights as the mother. If this happens the father must assert his rights to stay with and hold the baby so that some bonding can take place.
>
> *This is a HUGE part of Natural Childbirth!*
> *Refuse that offer to "Take something for the pain"!*

First Breastfeeding

It is truly amazing that some babies will suck as though really hungry … in fact, starving. Only a few minutes old and acting like a pro! Other babies are less interested, but all babies will nuzzle and search for the nipple. Touch your baby's cheek and watch the reaction. He immediately turns to that side with mouth open. They are born with that automatic reflex to find food. As your nipple becomes erect from the baby's touch, your uterus will contract and help the placenta to be expelled and the lining of the uterus to remain tight. A tight, hard, contracted uterus will prevent excessive bleeding.

The sooner you get your baby to breast, the better for your body and your baby. They belong together still!

It is about this time that the doctor will inject a local anesthetic into the edges of your episiotomy, if you had one, or your tear if that happened. When the local has made you numb, and you are busy fussing over your sweet new baby, the doctor will then begin to "embroider" the edges of your cut or tear together. You do not have to worry about the drug getting to your baby at this point.

During this time, the placenta may be expelled. This is called the third stage of labor and may require a push from you. Anytime up to 30 minutes is perfectly normal for the placenta to be delivered. Having the baby at breast usually facilitates the third stage.

When all these details have been completed, you'll be padded (there will be considerable bloody vaginal discharge) and cleaned up a bit. The bed will be restored to its normal position and you will be able to sit up and become comfortable. Your job is finished for the day! Congratulations!

Expect to have orange juice offered to you … it's one of the rewards—you need some sugar in you to replenish your energy that has been used in the past few hours. Of course, your husband, coach, partner—whoever has worked hard along with you throughout your labor has earned a glass of juice as well. Consider it a toast to the new baby! Well done!

Immediately After Birth

If the labor was a normal one, and you and your doctor agree, you may now walk about to stretch your legs. At some point you will need to go to bed for a good sleep, but the excitement will keep you going for a while. You will be watched very carefully for blood pressure, pulse and bleeding for two hours. The nurse will check the tightness of your uterus and if it loosens, she'll "knead" it into a tight contraction again. Not comfortable but necessary. You can help by massaging and kneading it yourself. Ask the nurse to show you exactly how to do it effectively. Sometimes you will be given an ice bag to put on your tummy to help the process. It is important that your uterus remain firm, so that there will not be bleeding from the detachment of the placenta from the lining of the uterus. That's why breastfeeding is such a bonus at this stage. It causes a contraction of the uterine muscles.

Hopefully, the baby will be left with you throughout as much of this period as possible. There is increasing evidence that these immediate moments after birth are important to the baby. The stimulus of your touch is important to even his breathing and heartbeat. Much is happening in that tiny being, and the closeness to you, the mother, can help it to be smooth and easy.

> *During the first two hours, try to nurse, nuzzle, cuddle, stroke and love your baby all you can. This bonding will last his and your lifetimes.*

For these two hours, you will be very excited. You want to shout to the world about your new baby. Your husband will brag about you, how well you did, how beautiful you are, how sweet the baby is. It's especially fun to phone the grandparents to announce the new arrival. With today's video capabilities and smartphones, a photo of your little one has probably already been beamed around the world.

No one will believe that you could have just had a baby and sound so well and happy. And look so good! Our society has warped this whole business of childbirth. In the old days, the new mother was bed-ridden for a week or more. Now, she's up and about right away … yet understands that there is some healing needed. Today's new mother will take care of herself as well as her baby. It starts with the simple movement of walking around, getting nourishment and then resting.

Therefore:

After two hours of excitement . . .

Hyperactive laughing and talking . . .

Holding and admiring the baby . . .

Trying to breastfeed . . .

Photographing and videoing . . .

Phoning friends and relatives to share your grand news . . .

Being famished and finding a snack . . .

Trying to adjust to your new roles as parents . . .

 Finally you will begin to lose some of your energy . . .

It's time for a long, long deserved good sleep—you've earned it . . .

Make sure you keep your newborn nearby as you sleep. You will rest better . . .

Listen to your own body. Don't let others tell you how you feel—whether they are a doctor, nurse, spouse, partner, coach or best friend. Listen to your body and act on your own instincts. You know what is best for you.

You just proved it by having a Natural Childbirth!

What if the Baby is Breech?

In the past, doctors would work with the mothers if a baby was in the breech position or any position other than the head coming down the birth canal first. In most cases, the baby would be delivered vaginally and usually in one push. That's changed dramatically today. Rarely is a breech baby born without a Caesarean Section. In fact, few OBs have been taught or know how to do it the "old fashion way." Why?—there is a risk involved ... and litigation if things go wrong.

If your baby hasn't turned position prior to labor starting, most doctors just schedule your delivery as a Caesarean—setting the birth date—you have little choice.

Here's what I would do if I knew my baby was in the breech position:

1. Ask—is there a doctor in your city who does Vaginal Breech Births?

2. Ask—is there anyone in the community who works with mothers in turning babies prior to delivery? It's often successful and certainly worth a try. There is a Chiropractic Technique which has been successful.

3. Ask—does the hospital or birthing center have specific rules if a baby presents breech?

4. Ask—does the doctor have a set policy for dealing with babies that present breech?

5. Ask—will your doctor allow the mother to go into labor before scheduling surgery?

Why? … Because being in labor is good for your baby. The contractions stimulate the body in preparation for birth.

A little squeezing by the uterus stimulates the nervous system to prepare your baby to get ready for the new life he will encounter in just a short time.

Ask your doctor why the Caesarian Section needs to be scheduled at a time and date that has not been determined by either your body or the baby. As far as I know, science has not yet determined exactly what causes the body of the mother to produce the specific balance of hormones that gets the labor to begin. Don't be surprised if you meet a great deal of resistance from the doctor. Caesarian sections are scheduled to fit the calendar of the hospital and the doctor. Otherwise it has to be scheduled as an emergency surgery. I do not know why that is not acceptable to the medical professionals. Going into labor indicates that the baby is ready to be born and that should be a deciding factor on the birth date.

Put this in your Birth Plan to ask about the procedure used if the Breech position becomes a problem for you at the end of your pregnancy. At least you will know the possibilities and options or lack of them!

A Caesarean would certainly not be a first choice for any of us who plan for Natural Childbirth: after all, it is major surgery. It complicates the lovely "new mother" part of childbirth because of the use of anesthetic and analgesic drugs. You become a mother who does not feel well, and has a very sore tummy. You will have a longer time in the hospital. You have a right to be disappointed but accept what can't be changed! If a surgical birth becomes a necessity, then concentrate on the outcome—a beautiful, healthy baby. Enjoy your reward!

Rhondda's Tip

The Baby is so ready to meet and greet you! It is amazing how she will look directly into your eyes and lock into your soul! You cannot tear your eyes away!

Do not wait! As soon as you can reach your baby slide her up onto your tummy, amniotic fluid, blood and all and let her slither up to your breasts. Feel the lovely contact between you. So sensual! The father, too, can participate, massaging and stroking both of you, rubbing the natural lubricant into the skin of all three of you as he welcomes his child into the world.

What a different world it is! Imagine coming from the security of the warm, dark, watery capsule to the cool, bright, dry air. The change is staggering … noise, touch, smells, harsh light, bright vision, making sounds for the first time, using her lungs to breathe, swallowing your milk. The newness of it all! Your smell and sound must be the only familiar aspect of this new world. That alert, sensitive, tiny being is taking it all in during the first few minutes of life. Make her feel welcome!

When she becomes tired of absorbing it all and takes her nap she will be secure, safe and assured that the one part she recognizes is still there with her … Mother.

Chapter 19

Parenthood

Now you two are parents! You concentrated so hard on having the baby that perhaps you did not put a lot of time into thinking about your new roles as being a Mom and Dad. Most likely, you've had some discussion on what sort of parents you want to be, but have you done anything more than make pronouncements such as "My kid won't …" or, "I'm certainly not going to allow …"?

This is serious business. You have a built-in pattern of parenting from your own parents. Do you want to be that same parent? Rarely have I had a new mother tell me that she would raise her child exactly the way her parents raised her. Most likely, you will want to change some aspects! Unfortunately, it's a hard pattern to change. Parenting is often more emotional than you intend.

To enlarge your ideas of becoming parents, you might begin a "New Parent Group" and meet with the members of your Bradley Method childbirth-training class to discuss being parents. This could be just mothers and babies or a couples group. It would be a forum for exploring your values and ideas with others. You would be a support for one another. You will learn from each other. La Leche League will give you involvement with other parents, also. Do it as a couple or separately but do explore your options in preparing for parenting.

I know that being a La Leche League Leader made me a much better mother than I could have been without the examples of the mothering of other breastfeeding mothers. There is a comfortable and natural style to mothering that seems to come with the ease of breastfeeding the baby. It was satisfying to have others to follow, watch and copy as I learned to be a mother. As a group we would discuss our problems and how we solved them. I learned early what it means in the saying, "It takes a village to raise a child." If you have a strong, friendly support group it will be your village.

You may already have your village! I did not. If you live near your family and many friends whom you've known for years, you have your village already made. If you are living far away from your family and close friends then you need to build that strong support group.

You and your mate will fall into fewer bad habits of parenting if you continue to discuss your values as parents as your child grows. I feel that each generation has the responsibility to improve the quality of life for its children to some degree. You'll do that with good parenting. If you believe that you had good parenting, then emulate that and try to be even better. If you were less than satisfied with the way you were treated as a child, then make sure that you change that pattern with your own children. Just because it was your upbringing doesn't mean that it has to pass on to your child. It is not easy but it will be worth it in your child's life.

There are many good books and other sources of information which I hope you will pursue. Don't take for granted that you will be the perfect parent that you want to be. You will not! You are a victim of your own emotions. You have bad days and good. Who doesn't? Some things will upset you for reasons not even consciously known to you. It is amazing that your child comes to you with a personality built in! Didn't your mother warn you that you could have a child exactly like you?

There are so many variables. Richard frequently said to our oldest son Joe, when he became old enough to complain about some fatherly rule, "I'm doing my best, Joe. Remember that I've never before been a father." As a matter of fact, Richard was a fantastic father, and I believe that his success secret is in the statement of his wise words above. He treated each child with respect and love and each experience on its own merits. He tried to be consistent but was not afraid to be flexible.

Being consistent with children is the biggest myth in our culture. It leads to, "Because I said so" parenting. Flexibility is far more important than being consistent! Think through each event and deal with it on its own merits.

Children, even babies, respond very well to honesty. Those are the standards Richard and I set as parents—respect and honesty. We felt very strongly the awesome responsibility of our role as parents and hoped that our children would go into the world able to cope with life and experience happiness and fulfillment. Now I am able to reap the rewards of realizing that we did raise five children who have become outstanding adults. They exemplify the values and qualities that make me proud. Also I like to be with them! They are my best friends and give me loyal, loving support—something that I think is one of the true benefits of successful parenting.

When I was a young mother, my husband and I became interested in a book about parenting, *Parent Effectiveness Training* by Thomas Gordon. He described a very different way of treating children than was commonly used when our kids were young, but it appealed to us. Without knowing this, my daughter and her husband attended a class on this very same book after they had children. They liked the ideas presented and in fact began using it as a basic philosophy to raise their own children. My daughter, Claryss Nan Jamieson, is now a teacher of the classes and has co-written a workbook based on the same principles, *Teaching Parents a Guidance Approach*, by Jamieson, Porter and Sellery.

Begin now to explore your ideas about being parents. This is not a skill that "just comes naturally." You will learn as you go but begin the learning as soon as possible. It will be surprising to you how differently you think from your mate. You have been raised with some different values. These differences need to be explored and evaluated early. Raising a child does not always bring a couple closer together. It could very well divide you. Do we think about this when we are in the early stages of falling in love and then deciding to have a baby? Of course not! Now that you are about to become a family this has meaning for you.

Now that I've discussed philosophy of parenting with you, let's get back to that beautiful newborn baby.

The Challenge of a Newborn Baby

The good news is that a new born infant sleeps a great deal. It is not unusual for it to be 20 hours a day. There is very little crying at first. Unfortunately, that does not last for long! It allows you a chance to get some rest in the first few weeks—although it's not an eight hour stretch—a few hours here, and a couple there. Brand new babies also sleep very soundly. For about two or three months, you do not have to be quiet with a newborn. Noise does not waken them. As they get older, this does change and parents are frantic to keep a baby sleeping. Waking their child is a federal offense!

A crying baby is a challenge to you. Is he wet? Is he hungry? Does he need burping? Is anything sticking him? Is his position uncomfortable? Try one possible solution after another until your baby is secure again. Perhaps he simply needed your touch. He's been in constant contact with you for nine months. Is it any wonder that he cries when he wakens alone in a hard, dry, cold bed? He must miss your soft, wet, warm uterus! Pick your baby up in your arms and cuddle him. Once the baby has stopped crying, he may actually be hungry. Just because the nursing was refused at the beginning do not accept that it is not what he wants now that the crying has stopped. Try again.

Crying Is the Baby's Way of Asking for Help

Please do not worry about "spoiling" your baby. You can indulge an older child, and he may become an unhappy and unpleasant little creature, but you can't spoil a tiny child with love and cuddling. It is perfectly normal and OK for a baby to cry. It's not OK for you to ignore his cry in the ridiculous attempt to "not spoil" him! Your baby will cry sometimes when you cannot get to him for a few minutes but he should have the security of knowing that his cry will be answered. Can you imagine the hopelessness of a baby whose only means of calling for help is ignored?

When a baby cries, he has a need. Most likely, when you fulfill the need your baby will stop crying. Respect his need for help. He has no other way to communicate. You begin that very first day of your child's life by respecting him as an individual with his own very specific needs.

There may be times when you honestly can't solve the problem. You try every way you know how and the baby cries. You know he's not sick; you've fed, changed, checked, walked, burped, sung to, danced with and rocked him. You still have a crying baby. (A rare case, it is true.) By now you begin to lose perspective. It's easy to feel that the baby is no longer respecting you!

At this point, it's time to call Daddy to help. "Save me from my child," is a valid need on the part of the mother. Amazingly, the baby may settle down right away with a calm father. If the father is not home, you could take a walk outside with baby in his carriage. Go to a neighbor's for coffee—or be honest with her and go for help!

Some of you do not have a 'Daddy' to call for rescuing. Make sure you have at least one person you can call on the phone, to ask for help. You could ask her over for coffee or just to visit for a few minutes. Become close enough friends that you could call her at midnight if you needed her. Perhaps there is another new mom in your neighborhood or apartment building who would like to be a Baby Buddy. You could take turns with the babies when either of you needs rest. Take an afternoon walk together. It would refresh any mother who is in an overwhelmed state. If you stroll down the street alone with your baby in the carriage, you'll make a new friend! It is lovely that human beings of all ages respond to babies as they do.

Babies sometimes have a tummy ache. In fact I now know from experience that some babies have tummy aches a lot! All the rocking and singing and nursing and loving and crooning and dancing that can possibly be given by kind loving parents does not always cure the crying. This is when you need a support group to help you or a grandmother to come to help. At least that validates you. Your baby is not telling you that you are a lousy mother when even grandmother cannot stop the crying. After you have had the baby checked by the doctor and there seems to be nothing medically wrong, you will try everything that friends and medics tell you to do. When nothing seems to help consistently, you have faith that gradually it will get better … and it does! All you can do is continue to love and cuddle your baby through those times.

Do not be surprised if you have emotional ups and downs in moods. Your body is going through a very big change in these postpartum days and you may find yourself crying over small things that really do not matter ... burned biscuits ... or "someone" left the milk out overnight. I plead with that new father for just a bit of extra patience. It will help you a lot if you get sympathy and understanding. Raging hormones is not an exaggeration. After ten days or two weeks, you should be more like yourself again.

You may need extra help with constant and inconsolable crying. It can really get on your nerves! Do not blame the baby. Do not punish the baby. If you find yourself getting angry with the baby—call for help, reach out, and find someone to rescue you. Put your baby in a safe place in a comfortable position with every need filled to the best of your ability then leave the baby with someone else and go where you cannot hear the crying. Call someone to come to help you. A friend that is close by, or even a soothing voice on the phone that tells you that you are OK will help to calm you. A crying baby is very nerve wracking and can make you feel very angry and irrational. Believe me you are not alone in this experience. It is extremely important that you do not try to handle this on your own. You need help and support. This is when you need your village.

There are times when you simply do not know what to do. You feel an utter failure as a mother. You need someone to rescue you. That is when you need help and MUST have someone you could call to take over for you.

Let's face it—your hormones may be way out of balance—if the crying is getting on your nerves, causing you to feel upset, it makes sense to call your doctor.

"After baby blues" is not a rarity—it's much more common than most mothers admit to. If you feel that your baby is crying a lot and if you feel that you are ready to punish your child for the crying, then it is time to get help. Determine if it's anything physical, something you can correct, for either you or your baby. If not, make that phone call. First call a support friend or family member to come to rescue you before you do something hurtful to your darling baby. Second, call your healthcare provider. It's part of your safety plan—for both you and your baby.

Most of us experience a short period of "after baby blues" so if you ask, you will get support from other mothers when you are going through this. It is usually short lived if you can get some supportive help, lots of rest, good nourishing food and make sure you are not taking any medication. If you have been told to take pills for pain or any drugs for any reason, that could be the cause of your "blues." If it continues after a week or two then you need serious help from your doctor. We mothers all think that we can rise above all our difficulties … don't be too proud to ask for help.

Remember you must:

- Get lots of sleep and rest.
- Get friendly and sympathetic help and support.
- Get nourishing food and regular meals.
- Get off all drugs and have medications checked for depressing effects.

These are all things that friends and family will do for you. But you have to ask. No one can help you if they do not know what you are going through. Accept that you might need help with this new experience in your life.

Begin your plan now. Bring this to the attention of the Bradley Method Class that I insist you find. Discuss the idea of forming a support "go for help" friendship that you will maintain for after the baby is born, you all have a common need so use it to advantage.

221

When Is a Cry a Real Cry?

That first day, after you've rested, you may be overprotective of your baby. He will make "mewing" noises as he moves in his sleep, but don't disturb him. When he really needs you, he will cry. It will be a funny noise, but unmistakably a cry. Before many days, you'll begin to know the various kinds of cries he makes. It's different for his various needs. A frantic baby will make a frantic cry. And there will be an "I'm beginning to be hungry" cry. There are many others such as:

I'm wet and need changing.

I need to burp.

I'm afraid.

I need to know you are nearby.

I'm bored.

I want to play.

I'm lonely.

I hear you talking and want to join you.

I can't see because the blanket is covering my eyes … and so on!

You and your child will develop a close communication very quickly. When you have a busy, mixed-up day, do not expect the baby to be quiet and peaceful. Your emotions are too apparent to a breastfed baby. So listen carefully to his cries to figure out what he is telling you.

When the baby is a month or six weeks old, you will need to return to your health care provider for a postpartum checkup. Find out when you are expected to have an appointment. You will be examined vaginally to determine your return to normal. Now you may consider yourself ready for any activity you choose!

Rhondda's Tip

What I want to say to you young mothers is—don't be ashamed of not knowing how. None of us knows how in the beginning. We learn gradually and there's no right and wrong. Every mother where you live would love to offer help. That's what mothers do best. Be humble enough to ask for help when you really need it. You'll make a friend because she'll be flattered. And what woman would not love to have a chance to hold and cuddle your newborn?

Chapter 20

Now You Are a Mother

Little did you know that getting pregnant was the beginning of a new Career!

W hen you decided to have a baby ... or discovered you were pregnant ... you did not realize that everything in your life was going to have to shift to make room for this new addition. You thought life would go on as usual with the lovely new being as a part of normal living. Now you are seeing that there is a shift going on regarding "normal." All this talk about nursing and not sleeping and crying and crying a lot is like an earthquake in your life! Although I've introduced the idea of major changes for you, I hope you've been remembering the lovely new mother part that I've also shared with you. I want to be positive but want you to be aware of the possible problems as well. So back to your preparation for being the best mother in the whole wide world! To be the good mother you want to be, you need stimulation of some kind. The mother who has a job will have that but will be frustrated that her mothering time is too short. The mother who quits work to be a full-time mother must seek outside diversions because she is not used to being alone in her home with no adult communication.

How do you deal with these problems? I've found that it helps to divide your needs into physical, emotional, social and intellectual.

Physical ... Get the Body Moving

There are so many options for exercise! It is all a matter of making it a priority. Walking is always available and free. So is using an exercise program on TV or internet.

I have found that if I join a group, I am more likely to do it. Find a way to get total body exercises that will keep your figure in shape and keep you feeling energized. Most communities have very good fitness programs for a nominal amount of money. If you pay for a class you'll be less likely to skip. Many adult classes have nursery arrangements, too. Any community will have privately taught dance or fitness classes. Modern dance, Pilates and ballet are marvelous for figure and self-image. Yoga is very popular and you can find classes most anywhere. Make it a priority in your life.

You could organize your own program. Invite several friends—or even one—to join you and get a DVD of your choice to give the exercise you want. Make it a regular and a definite commitment so that you will get a worthwhile workout, TV offers great exercise programs, an endless variety, too. It's always more fun if you have a friend or a group and can exercise together. Take bike hikes, play tennis or go swimming. Exercise stimulates your circulation so that you feel invigorated, think better and have more energy. Your life long health depends on it. It is never too early to take responsibility for your own health and wellbeing. You will be a better mother if you feel good about yourself.

Learn New Skills and Get Social

You also need to be stimulated intellectually. You cannot stay at home all day—every day—with a baby who does not talk and expect to be a scintillating conversationalist when you are with your friends. You need to talk about something other than your baby, fascinating as that is to the baby's father and the grandmother! What young full-time mother of one or more small children does not feel the need for something exciting, grown-up and intellectual in her life at least once in a while?

If you are a stay-with-the-baby mother by choice then it is up to you to make it a fun time in your life. You have chosen to stay at home and devote these years to your children. Now you must be creative to satisfy your need for an interesting life while you are a mother. You must choose activities that are interesting and exciting and that fit in with your joy of being a mother. Become thoughtful about this and start a list of all the activities you think might be fun to learn or skills you'd like to develop. It will be your Bucket List!

Anything goes! How about enrolling in a course on psychology at the local college, or joining a book group at the library? The possibilities of classes to take and groups to join are endless. Whatever you have an urge to do or to study or to learn—now is the time.

The wonderful and awful thing about having a baby is that most of the friends you spend time with are not having babies at the same time as you! If they do happen to be mothers or pregnant, then it could strengthen your friendship. On the other hand you may find that your interest in Natural Childbirth and Breastfeeding might not be shared by your friends and in fact you could be judged for it negatively. Also, their pattern of parenting will greatly affect your friendship if you don't agree with them. So ... It is a good time in life to make a few new friends! The friends that I made during that time in my life are generally still my very dear friends.

Being a full time mother has some definite advantages. Your day is yours to plan. Naps and feeding are fairly flexible with babies and young children. You develop a tolerance for "child-noise" and can concentrate despite it. Sometimes you can arrange a baby-sitter or nursery situation to fit your needs. You have no valid excuse for not doing things you want to do. Find new friends to share new ideas with you.

Or you may be so happy and so content and so fulfilled in your new role as a mother that you do not want to do anything else. That is marvelous. As long as you are satisfied with your life, don't try to change it. However, you will find that even a walk in the park with your baby will bring new people and experiences into your life. Babies are magnets! It will keep your life interesting.

I channeled my energies into childbirth teaching as soon as Joe was born and it has been a perfect solution for me. I taught one or two evenings a week, when Richard could baby-sit and usually I took the newest breast feeding baby with me.

As well as teaching these classes, I became a leader of La Leche League. These were evening meetings in my own home and only once a month. There's no better way of meeting friends, feeling content and helping others. Along with that, I began going to a once-a-week class in modern dancing, took mandolin lessons and swimming lessons. Very quickly I had expanded to the point where I was too busy and needed to spend more time at home keeping things in order. I am a firm believer in arranging my time so that my family comes first. When I had young children they made sure that I did keep them a priority!

If you are devoting many years of your life to being a mother, you must also be a fulfilled individual. Do what is necessary to maintain your own self-image. Let me warn you about waiting until your children are in school to do all those things you want to do. You think you will have all day to yourself to do anything you choose. Sorry, it is not so!

When our five children were all in school, I had no more spare time than I ever had. It is different mothering, but not less busy. From my perspective now, my message remains unchanged! I never have time to fill—I only have time to fit things into my life that I want to do. Do not wait! In our family, we have a motto:
If not now ... when?

Children have a way of filling your time as they get older. Different mothering but not easier! Certainly no less busy! Never the less, it is the best job I have ever had! I have spent the rest of my life searching for something that was as rewarding and fulfilling as my career as a mother … nothing comes even close!

You may decide that you need to be working again. Then that is what you should do. If you have worked hard to be successful in your chosen profession you have the right to maintain that success. Perhaps it is a financial decision for you and you need to get back to your work to support the family.

The challenge for you is a very different one from the stay at home mom. You will be in conflict about leaving your baby with someone else to be the caretaker. Use your maternity leave to enjoy being the full time mom for as long as it lasts. Get breast feeding to a good schedule so that you will be able to continue feeding the baby even when you are not handy. There are several good sources of help in this, too—check my website, *www.NaturalChildbithExercises.com*. Whatever your reason for going back to work, it is up to you to make it as easy as you can for you and the baby.

Here is my formula for being a happy fulfilled mom who loves her job:

+ Keep your body fit.

+ Learn new skills.

+ Make new friends.

+ Maintain an interest in the world around you.

+ Love and cuddle that baby with all your being!

The simple truth of being a mother is that your child will always be the center of your world.

Rhondda's Tip

Becoming a mother is a culture shock for many. Everything is new and different and you begin to wonder who ... and sometimes what ... you are. You are tired. You are sleep deprived. You encounter emotional roller coasters. You have demands upon you that you never really imagined. Don't forget there is a YOU ... a you that also has to be nurtured and needs some care.

Chapter 21

After the Baby Tune-Up ... Postpartum Exercises

You've gotten your baby off to a terrific start, now it's time to focus on you. Throughout your pregnancy, you used a variety of exercises to assist you through your labor and delivery. Post-delivery, I am introducing exercises that will not only restore your body but create more energy for you physically and mentally.

Mabel Lumm Fitzhugh's postpartum exercises are some of my favorites. These marvelously effective exercises are specific for that part of you which was stretched out of shape while you were pregnant. They do not require very much energy so they are perfect for the first six weeks postpartum (after delivery of the baby). During this time, you should also be doing at least 80 pelvic rocks each day to get the uterus into the correct position in your body as it becomes firm and tight again.

You may have a vaginal discharge for up to six weeks. It's bloody for the first ten days or so and then becomes a dark brown. It is drainage from the healing uterus and is very normal.

I often forget to mention "after-birth pains," which are just what it says. They are a minimal problem with Natural Childbirth deliveries. For up to five days after the birth, you will feel the uterus as it contracts back down to its normal size. The contractions may be very strong and quite unpleasant. Your doctor will probably give you a stronger-than-aspirin type of drug to take if you need it. As a breastfeeding mother you do not want those drugs in your milk and on to the baby ... right? Do these exercises instead!

By coincidence, I discovered that the postpartum exercises relieved the worst afterbirth pains that I ever had. However, even with our fifth, Rich, my uterus contracted with so little pain that I was never tempted to take any medication. It is generally expected that after-birth pains are worse with each baby. If you are uncomfortable, try the postpartum exercises before resorting to any medication.

Throughout *Natural Childbirth Exercises*, I have given you postures and exercises for pregnancy—plan to incorporate them into your daily life forever!

Lifetime Exercises:

+ Pelvic rocks should be done every day. At least eighty will do. Before bed is still the best time and on hands and knees. It will keep your uterus in the proper place, your abdominal muscles firm and keep your back strong.

+ Standing pelvic rock has taught you to maintain that perfect posture. Use it always.

+ Tailor sitting is still the best possible sitting position—pregnant or not.

+ Squatting makes sense when you must get to the floor to reach anything. Now that you are not pregnant, you may want to use your legs to come up and not tip your body forward. It's up to you.

+ Kegels must be maintained throughout life for all the reasons given previously—twenty per hour while you are awake.

+ Use the relaxation techniques to make your life more peaceful. It helps when you are under stress. Don't forget, relaxation works well for your husband and children. You will find all sorts of times to use it. My adult kids still fondly remember being relaxed with these techniques at bedtime when they were children. Try it ... much better than be annoyed with them for not falling asleep on their own!

Below are the postpartum exercises I recommend for your post-baby tune-up. Use them all your life, too, whenever some tightening is needed.

Tummy-Tightener—Postpartum Exercise One

This will tighten all the parts of you stretched from your pregnancy. Your abdomen, thighs, Kegel, and bottom—the area of your body that needs to be returned to normal—will be tensed as you do this exercise. The rest of your body should have remained in good condition throughout your pregnancy, if you were maintaining reasonable exercise.

This is a good tummy-tightener for all women who have lost the muscle tone in their abdomen.

HOW:

To start, lie flat on your back. Cross your legs at the knees and put your hands on your abdomen. Now tighten in four ways:

1. Roll both knees toward each other, tightening the inner thigh. Hold.

2. Do a Kegel. Hold.

3. Raise your head until you feel your abdominal muscles tighten under your fingers. Hold.

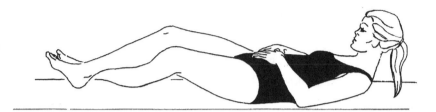

4. Squeeze your buttocks. Hold.

5. Release everything and relax.

Now repeat. Each of you will have your own "required" number of times. Some women have done it one hundred times a day and really look great. If ten a day keeps you firm, then that is fine. Perhaps it will take more or less, but find your own maintenance requirement.

WHERE:

All you need is a flat surface. You may lie on your bed, or a carpeted floor.

WHEN:

Have eight hours sleep after the baby is born and then begin a few postpartum exercises. No, you do not have to do that! It would not hurt you to do it but you will not be thinking about exercise for a week or more! When you do begin, work very slowly so as not to make yourself stiff and sore. Space these exercises throughout the day at comfortable intervals. I suggest that you work up to twenty a day by six weeks after the baby is born. If you want to do more, that is fine.

When I have been lazy and my abdominal muscles get loose and flabby, I do ten to fifty of these daily—plus the next postpartum exercise, which goes with it—and in two days I can tell the difference. It really works and fast! The beauty of these exercises is that they can both be done as you go to bed at night because they are easy and quiet and you'll be able to fall asleep afterward (when can't a new mother fall asleep?). They do not necessarily invigorate you, as so many exercises do. Sometimes I forget to exercise until I am in bed at night, so these are a blessing.

Waist Trimmer—Postpartum Exercise Two

This exercise, specifically for the waist and midriff as well as the abdomen, is the completion of the first postpartum exercise. The two should always be done together.

This will help you button your waistbands again!

HOW:

1. Lie flat on your back on a padded floor. Bend one knee slightly—about four inches from the bottom of your knee to the floor.

2. With the opposite hand, point toward the raised knee. Your head is raised and your one shoulder. You can feel the pull through your waist.

3. Relax.

4. Bend the other knee slightly and point toward it with the opposite hand and shoulder.

5. Relax.

6. Do at least 10 times each side, more if you wish.

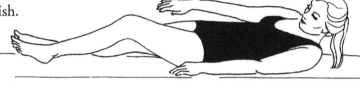

If you can touch your knee with your hand, you are a contortionist, or your arms are very long, or most likely, you have your knee raised too high!

WHERE:
On the same surface as postpartum exercise one.

WHEN:
Immediately following postpartum exercise #1, Tummy Tightener.

Rhondda's Tip

There is a new you with a new baby in your life. Most mothers strive to get back into shape—whatever that shape is envisioned to be. These simple post partum exercises will get you on your path without adding stress to your already complicated day.

Chapter 22

Rhondda's Final Words

I have no illusions that this book is an "everything you ever wanted to know about Natural Childbirth," it is not! It is a primer to get you started on the most amazing experience of your life.

The writing of this book has been a compulsion for me. Years ago, I started the project of revising my book that is out of print, *Exercises for True Natural Childbirth* written as a companion book to Dr. Bradley's *Husband Coached Childbirth*. It was written at his urging.

In this writing I had many starts and stops along the way. My life changed; my children turned into adults; weddings (five of them); grandchildren (nine); other careers for me: Real Estate, Masters Degree, Healing Touch; travel; and becoming a widow (Oh My!). During all of this busy, fulfilling life, I kept coming back to my need to rewrite my book. I loved being a published author but I did not like to write. Nevertheless, I felt that I had experience, expertise and exercises that I need to share with new mothers.

Then I met Judith Briles, an author of over 30 books and a motivator beyond my wildest dreams. She took me into her fold, used her expertise and with her shepherding, my miracle of a published book has come into your hands.

The process of explaining to others what my book is about and why I would be writing it has brought me into focus on what Natural Childbirth is and how important it has been in my life. I began a search into myself to understand what makes some of us embrace it and others to find it abhorrent. I began asking myself, what do we bring to it and what do we receive from it? To you I share my wisdom on the matter.

Natural Childbirth is not just about having a baby

It is about living your life.

It is about *responsibility*. Taking it or giving it away.

It is about choices, conviction and completion.

Rhondda's Kernel of Truth:

I know that to have a Natural Childbirth without drugs you must take *responsibility* for it yourself. You cannot expect anyone else to do it for you. Not your coach; not your doctor; not the hospital's staff; and not me nor this book. You, and only you, can make it happen. You cannot simply *let* it happen, you must *make* it happen.

When you choose Natural Childbirth, you take *responsibility* for:

Your pregnancy

The birth

No drugs during the birth

The outcome

Your body

Your health

Your baby

Your family as a Mother

This is not just about the birth, not just breastfeeding, not just exercising, not just about having the best coach, not just about diet and eating well, not just bonding with the baby, not just being a good mother and wife … No! It is about taking *responsibility* for your whole life.

None of us makes the right choices all the time. Some of our wishes in life are not granted. Accept the circumstances. Do not be a victim. Do not blame others for your failures. Do not seek sympathy. Do not seek revenge.

Accept the failure life has thrown at you, accept it, learn from it, and get on with your life.

Not all childbirths are storybook perfect. There are many factors involved. The environment is a factor; stress; DNA comes into play; some mothers slip and misuse drugs and alcohol; you might even catch the measles or the flu. There are a variety of happenings, often unexpected, that can and will affect a pregnancy and birth. We may not like the outcome but we must accept it.

You can blame others, you can blame circumstances, you can blame your doctor or your childbirth educator and you can even blame your body. But don't be a victim. Accept the experience, learn from it, find some good in it and realize it is still your responsibility. Accept the *responsibility* for your life, create it, and make it happen. If you are thrown a curve, move around it and keep on with the best solution.

I thought I was writing this book to teach you about Natural Childbirth, to let you know how important it is to do the exercises to prepare your body; and for a birth without drugs to protect your baby's brain from the harm that they cause. I hope I have done all that. But the idea of *responsibility* kept repeating in my head.

None of us makes the right choices all the time.

What makes you think that Natural Childbirth is what you want?

What makes you know that you are going to breastfeed your baby?

Could it be that these are normal functions for your body?

Could it be that it is the right thing to do and your body is ready and able to do what it is intended to do?

I have lived with my choice of Natural Childbirth for a long time now. I've had enough years to look back over my life and recognize how my choices have influenced and woven through my life.

To choose Natural Childbirth is to say:

Let me do it myself.

I can do it by myself; you do not need to do it for me.

Teach me how so I can do it on my own.

Let it not be done to me or for me.

I will make it happen.

Help me, instruct me, coach me, support me, tell me my mistakes but let me do it.

To have Natural Childbirth, attitude is always an essential ingredient. Your openness and positivity as you look forward to your birth will greatly enhance your journey through pregnancy.

As I have been going through the process of writing, I have learned a great deal about myself but more important is that I know a great deal about you, my dear reader.

Here is what I know about you:

> You are an independent woman.
>
> You are capable.
>
> You believe in yourself.
>
> You know, trust and respect your body.
>
> You are willing to be different and stand out in a crowd.
>
> You understand that it is normal and natural for your body to give birth.
>
> You are aware that pregnancy is a normal state of health, it is not a disease.
>
> You have strong beliefs and principles.
>
> You do not compromise your values.
>
> You fight for right.
>
> You like to be in control and you hate being out of control.

I also see you as a woman who is:

Passionate . . . Strong . . . Capable . . . Sensible . . . Smart . . . Thoughtful!

A woman who will take *responsibility* for your birth and your life!

Dear Mother-to-be,

I trust that your Birth will be exactly as you plan it to be and expect it to be.

The responsibility of birthing a baby is huge but you accept it with conviction and joyful anticipation,

knowing that you are ready for the challenge.

You are prepared with knowledge.

You are capable with a strong, *exercised*, healthy body.

You are excited to experience this amazing miracle of life.

You are joyful about becoming a Mother.

You accept and understand the *responsibility* of Natural Childbirth.

I admire and applaud you!

Congratulations.

My Love, Naturally,

Rhondda

Chapter 23

My Five Birth Stories

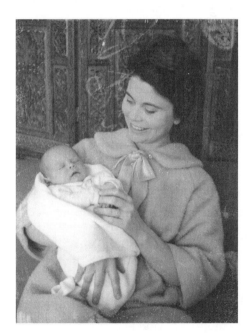

I have already warned you that women like to tell the details of the birth as it happened to them. In fact it seems to be a very great need on the part of all mothers. Does it surprise you then, that I am no different? I would like to tell about my five births just because I love to relive them, but I have another reason. I would like you to see that all five of my births were different. It will help you to see that even with that number it is hard to see them as the same or predictable. I want you to realize that when I seem to be unwilling to state facts about your expected birth it is because there is no predictability about how it will happen. I like to think that natural childbirth allows you choice in the experience. However, it seems to be largely up to the baby. Do you think that the mother really controls the birth or is it the baby … it is a conundrum!

Natural childbirth was about the furthest thing from my mind when I started my first job with my Bachelor of Science in Nursing from the University of Alberta, Canada. As a matter of fact, it was not a well-known idea. But five blooming young pregnant women came to me for help concerning natural childbirth as I started my public health career in the town of Lacombe, Alberta. Their conviction inspired me to help them.

My first approach was to go to their obstetrician for help but though he was very pleasant, he sent me on my way with a condescending "You're young yet, dear." I knew from nursing training how most births were conducted, that most doctors were in full control and delivered babies from a fully anaesthetized woman who woke up hours later asking if she'd had her baby yet.

My supervisor, to whom I went with all my problems, was much more helpful and armed me with her blessings, a birth atlas, Maternity Center Association Guides for Teaching, and a phonograph record by Dr. Grantly Dick-Read, recorded while his patients were in labor. To those five young women I owe my interest in childbirth training. We all learned a great deal together but we lacked a very important ingredient—experience. We all benefited nonetheless.

That was my introduction to natural childbirth. Little did I know how it was to affect the rest of my life. Next I moved to Montreal where I worked in a hospital and had no associations with pregnancy, so the subject of natural childbirth was not important to me again until I became pregnant myself.

Since nothing is more personal than childbirth experiences, and that is my subject, I think it only right to tell you something of how I met my husband.

My friend Mary Mulloy and I had saved and scrimped for a year and a half after graduation to buy steamship tickets to Europe. We went first to Portugal and Spain and spent a month touring before getting on another ship to cross the Mediterranean. It was on that ship I met Richard, a handsome, sophisticated lawyer from Denver, Colorado. It was love at first sight. After a chaotic, exciting, and romantic twelve days, our minds were made up (he took only five days, but I was more conservative), and six weeks after we met we were married in Switzerland in a small church on a daisy covered hill with the church bells ringing. There were eight of us including the bell ringer and an English-speaking minister. The next five months we spent honeymooning in Europe and Canada in a tiny Fiat car that we bought in Zurich. It was glorious. What's more, we never regretted our hasty decision!

The Birth Story of Joseph Baden

In the natural course of events I found my interest in natural childbirth was revived. In fact, by the time I introduced my husband to my parents, five months after we had married, I was also announcing their first grandchild was on his way! Soon after we settled into our apartment in Denver, Richard and I began to seek an obstetrician.

Richard had not given the birth process any thought and was puzzled when I announced we were going to have our child by natural childbirth. Even in a large major city, finding an obstetrician at that time who would know what "natural childbirth" meant required the services of a detective. Richard called his doctor friends, who scolded him for having such a foolish idea. Later, a nurse surreptitiously told him that to her knowledge there were only two doctors in the community who were sympathetic to the idea, Dr. Robert Bradley and his partner, Dr. Max Bartlett.

Sympathetic was the understatement of the century. They were wildly excited and enthusiastic! Our first appointment completely sold Richard, who, as an attorney, cross-examined Dr. Bradley for about an hour. The pregnancy began to take on new dimensions as every question was answered in a complete, intelligent, and sensible manner. We were not hurried and he gave us all the time we needed to ask questions. At the interview, we learned that these doctors:

1. Took as patients only couples who wanted natural childbirth.

2. Gave medication only with complications or if absolutely necessary. They never asked if you "wanted" it, as it was a medical judgment (6 percent were given anesthetic as a medical necessity.)

3. Had their office next door to the Porter Memorial General Hospital, so they could run across the street to "catch" a baby at any given time.

4. Gave five lectures and films to each couple in large groups.

5. Had six exercise classes taught by their own trained obstetrical Childbirth Educator. One year later that became me!

6. Expected husbands to share the total birth experience with their wives (including the birth) and would train them to coach their wives. This was unique. Nowhere else could a father attend the birth of his child in a hospital.

This was pure ecstasy. Suddenly, I had the full cooperation of the doctors and my husband as well. Exactly what I wanted. Richard became a salesman extraordinaire, convincing friends and neighbors, legal associates, and even strangers that they should use this sensible approach to having babies. The mystery, taboos, and magical aura were stripped away from the beautiful, functional thing that birth is meant to be.

Even a nurse does not know anything about being pregnant. I wanted to be told what was going on in my body. I liked the changes that were taking place as I practiced the simple postures and exercises that I was learning. It was fun to go to classes to learn about the strange changes that were taking place inside me. I was reassured to meet others in the classes that were sharing our experience with natural childbirth. We found that we liked the "natural childbirth" people!

Richard and I were having this extraordinary adventure together as a couple. It was so right, so important. He supported me and understood what was happening to me. He knew how important the exercises and postures were to the outcome of our birth. He accepted his role as coach and took it very seriously. Having our baby was not just woman's work. He became the coach, an important member of the team. A basic premise of Husband Coached Childbirth is that the father of the baby needs to be involved throughout pregnancy and the birth. I am sure it was important to the success of our marriage.

It became *our* pregnancy—an event which we shared and learned about and prepared for together!

Labor Begins

On April 1, the day before my due date, my body was surging with energy. I should have remembered about the "nesting" instinct, which is a term we've borrowed from animal behavior. When they sense the onset of labor, animals instinctively begin to prepare a nest for their young. A cat will frequently find clothes hamper and move the contents to a quiet, dark closet, working until she has a comfortable nest in which to give birth to her kittens. Nature seems to provide extra energy for all this activity. We human beings are apt to misuse the energy which nature provides at the beginning of our labor. In my case it happened to coincide with the day we moved from our studio apartment downtown, to a little three-bedroom house in the suburbs. Richard and I moved our entire personal belongings, and though there was not all that much, it took strenuous work to transport ourselves from apartment to home. I expended Herculean energy without difficulty, but was glad to crawl into bed about midnight.

Soon thereafter, I had a few contractions, but after carrying several tons of books what else could you expect? A little false labor, I thought. At 4 A.M., I was awakened with regular five-minute contractions. I walked around the house for about an hour to make sure they were real. Then we headed for the hospital.

In true new-father fashion, Richard, who had lived in Denver for ten years, lost his way to the hospital and approached panic in his need to get me safely to the doctor. He needn't have worried. The contractions continued at five minutes apart and I was barely dilated, with plenty of time for the usual procedure of hospital admittance.

I began my long vigil of relaxing with each contraction. Hurray! Hurray! It worked! Joy upon joy! All my fears and doubts about my own ability were quickly dispelled. All those nay-sayers could now be refuted. I was doing it and it worked as the doctor said it would. On and on I relaxed for twelve hours after coming to the hospital! Too bad that I had not recognized my "nesting instinct" and had saved that surge of energy for birth rather than moving, but it might have made no difference! The soon-to-be daddy was the one who became weary, and somewhat worried about the long labor. The medical staff reassured us that there was nothing to cause worry.

I do wonder how anyone can tolerate a labor without the calm, cool, and unhurried composure that relaxing and abdominal breathing give you. I was completely aware of the contractions, but was riding with them rather than fighting against them, and this was well worth the effort of the practicing I had done for all those months. I developed a new philosophy about a long labor; it is easier than a short fast labor because you have time to get very good at what you are doing! Whereas a fast labor might overwhelm you and never give you time to settle into the skill of relaxing with abdominal breathing.

The only disadvantage was my not being well rested before the onset of labor. However, I found that I could fall asleep between contractions, and then be roused by the next one enough to concentrate on relaxing, then back to snoozing again.

I did become somewhat edgy as transition into second stage arrived, and here Richard took over my relaxation. His calm, soothing voice would remind me to relax and breathe with my abdomen. He would remind me when to get ready for the next contraction and help me get relaxed with abdominal breathing as it was about to begin. He would count off the clock during a contraction so I would know how much longer it would last. It took great concentration and control during this part of labor. Without him during transition, natural childbirth might have gone down the drain!

In an instant the whole thing changed around. I couldn't relax nor did I want to relax anymore. The nurse advised that I should try one more relaxing contraction but it was not possible. The doctor stepped into the room and told me to go ahead and push. I had been holding my breath involuntarily.

Now we were into the exciting part of having a baby! My tiredness was gone. I felt peppy and happy. I was ready to work at this all night. How great it was to do something after all those hours of doing nothing. It was hard to do nothing but relax and breathe!

All the months of practicing holding my breath paid off. It was amazing to feel the tremendous tension begin to gather in the uterine area as I inhaled and expelled the first two breaths. Then I took my third big breath, held it, pulled my knees up to my shoulders, put my chin on my chest and pushed with all my might—then I felt nothing. No tension, No Pain. Nothing except good hard work and exhilaration. This is one time you cannot be ladylike. Don't be a weakling. It is now that you remember your pioneer ancestors and know that you are capable of intense physical effort. I put all my strength into each push and feelings of discomfort were gone. After several of these good hard pushes the doctor announced that he could see the baby's head. I was able to look in the mirror during the next push and could see a spot of black hair! His hair actually was blond but being wet it looked black!

It was time to move to the 'Delivery Room' as the concept of Birthing Rooms had not yet been discovered. By now I was feeling far too spunky and excited to be wheeled in on a bed so I advised the doctor that I would walk. He winked at a horrified nurse and we paraded out of the labor room down the hall into the room called Delivery.

The delivery room was more like a surgery room. The table was much like you see in the exam room at your doctor's office. The bottom of it drops and the head is adjustable. There are stirrups for your feet. Terribly unsatisfying for you but the doctor needs to be able to see what is going on! The good thing was that the head could be raised to nearly a forty-five degree angle to allow gravity to help your baby to slide down and out as you push. The doctor was sitting there to catch the baby.

Meanwhile Richard had changed to cap and gown and was sitting on a stool near the head of the table, ordinarily occupied by the anesthetist. His big role was to be the cheering section, as he mopped my brow with a sloshy wet cloth, which by the way felt glorious and he helped push my shoulders and head toward my chest to aid me in bearing down. I was very strong, our baby was very eager to be born, the coach was marvelous, and in a very short time I felt a sudden release. A flood of pleasure and sheer happiness swept through me: we had successfully completed the first nine months of our child's existence. My emotions led me to false conclusions, however, for I heard the doctor calmly say, "Now we have the head and with the next contraction we'll have the whole baby."

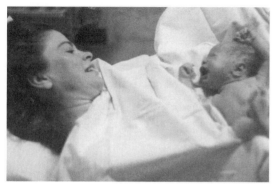

Waiting for the next push seemed to be an eternity, but it was a very short time, possibly two minutes. The last contraction took almost no effort, since the head is the largest part of the baby. The shoulders, then the rest of him easily arrived. What a miracle! What excitement! Proud papa realized he had a son and he shouted it for all to hear. "A boy, a boy, a boy!" We did have a boy name all ready, one from each grandfather, Joseph Baden.

This was such a happy time. There is nothing like it! Richard and I were talking excitedly while the doctor wiped and suctioned the loose mucus from the baby's tiny nose and mouth before he was placed on my now flat tummy. What a thrill to hold my own baby for the first time! Richard and I were laughing and crying together, proud and happy and thoroughly delighted with each other. At this opportune moment, the doctor injected some Novocain for the episiotomy repair. He had cut me during one of my pushes and I had not even known! It is startling how the pushing created numbness so that no anesthetic had been necessary. Now the pushing was all over, and I would certainly have felt the suturing! The local anesthetic was kindly given to me, as it could no longer harm the baby. By the time all this embroidering was done, the placenta was loosened and expelled. I would not have been aware of it except that the doctor, knowing we'd be interested, explained to us what was going on.

After changing to a fresh nightie, I was on my feet, proudly holding our new son in one arm, my other arm around my husband, both of us beaming with huge smiles. The doctor had now switched to his role as photographer, using our camera. I felt fantastically good. Walking was a relief after the strenuous work during the pushing.

251

In addition, I still had a vast amount of excited energy. The pride of my husband as he took my arm for the walk down the hospital corridor is one of my most precious memories.

Next stop was the recovery room. Remember this was a long time ago and we pioneers in Natural Childbirth had only begun to change the system. What a beautiful place to run up a huge telephone bill (no cell phones, either) calling everybody from coast to coast—California and Connecticut—and from top to bottom—Canada and Texas. Everyone had to know. New parents are generally insufferable, and we were perhaps the worst of the lot!

For a couple of hours, the nurses frequently checked my blood pressure, pulse, and uterus—to make certain it was contracted and hard. All things were normal. The baby was left in my arms during this time for us to love and admire. He even nursed a little. A three-day hospital stay was routine and since this was my first experience, I did go to a room in the maternity ward and was tucked into bed for the night. By this time it was 9 P.M. and I had done two days' work on a limited night's sleep. I was ready for a good rest. However, I awakened very early in the morning, before dawn, to listen to the birds and to contemplate my new role as a mother. What a timeless feeling it was to be carrying on the ancestral line and to be but a small fragment of eternity, and at the same time, the frightening weight on my heart of the responsibility I now held as the mother of a new life, a new individual unlike any ever known—unique and entirely different!

Joey and I spent two more days in the hospital. Everything went smoothly and the staff was very nice to me, but I was eager to get home and share our baby with Richard. We left for home with our precious bundle on the morning of my birthday. Of course, we stopped for a birthday lunch, cake and all, and the baby slept peacefully. I sat comfortably for more than an hour and wondered why there is so much fuss made about heat lamps and "stitches." This natural childbirth was paying dividends at every stage.

We were not very different from most new parents arriving home to the newly painted nursery. We held our baby between us, admired him, and asked each other, "What do we do now?" That did not last long as we launched into our new routine. I was breastfeeding, so that part was easily taken care of—though it took time. In fact, I spent all my time with my baby. Nothing else seemed very important. There was no time for anything else!

It was a continuous round of feeding, bathing, changing, rocking him to sleep. Before I could believe it, the baby was ready to be fed again. I gradually learned to manage everything but will never forget that period, and I do try to warn new mothers of it.

When Joey was six weeks old, I began training to teach for Dr. Bradley. I was truly gratified and honored to have been invited to become his Childbirth Educator. I began my new career along with new motherhood with great enthusiasm for both.

Claryss Nan

Being parents agreed with us and we could hardly wait to have another baby. Two years later, on March 1, Claryss Nan arrived. My labor began at a La Leche League meeting at the home of Mary Ann and Tom Kerwin. I called Richard to come and take me to the hospital. We were excited but also very relaxed and in control. I was comfortable moving about much longer into the labor than I had been with our first. Second-stage labor was different in that I was far more aware of the pressure of the baby against the perineum. Pushing was much faster this time and in no time we had delivered a beautiful "round-headed" girl. (Joey's head had been somewhat pointed, molded from the long labor.)

We were thrilled to have a girl. This time we had decided to do what the Kerwins had pioneered—come home right away with the baby. Mary Ann had home births in Chicago but Dr. Bradley was unwilling to do that. He had agreed to a happy compromise, however. A nursing baby and mother could be released from the hospital two hours after birth if there were no complications.

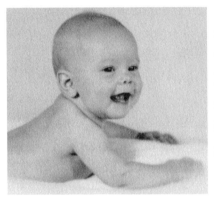

After two hours in the recovery room, during which time our pediatrician checked the baby, we proudly took Claryss Nan home to Joey, who was just waking up. He'd been asleep when I'd called Richard, so a sitter had been hired for the night. Grandmother Hartman had come out by taxi and the baby sitter was getting ready for school when we arrived home. Joey thought he'd never seen anything so marvelous as that baby. We all agreed. The best part of going home with the new baby was the reaction of her two-year-old brother.

I felt terrific after this birth. Comparing it to the first time, I now realized that I had been tired and a little shaky when I brought Joey home. I could not restrain myself this time! I invited people in for coffee and baby viewing and showed off in various ways. My poor neighbors were a bit dumfounded.

Second babies are such a joy. Claryss Nan was so good and my experience in mothering helped. We enjoyed our two children so much that it was inevitable that Rienne Frances would come along. She did on January 15—2 years later.

Rienne Frances

Rienne decided to announce her incipient arrival while I was conducting a La Leche meeting at my home. (My babies picked great company!) It was the only time my membranes ruptured in early labor. I'd had a few scattered contractions during the day but nothing definite. The meeting was over and we were visiting when suddenly I seemed to have no control and thought I was wetting my pants! I pulled my Kegel muscle as tightly as I could and it got me to the bathroom, where I realized what was happening. The last of the ladies left while Richard and I called a neighbor to come and baby-sit for the night. Claryss Nan must have sensed what was going on, for she woke up during our preparations and came into our bedroom as I was relaxing on the bed with a rather hard contraction. It disturbed her to see me take no notice of her so she pulled my eyelid open with her fingers. All that practice in relaxing was very important!

We were excited but did not break speed limits driving to the hospital. As I was being admitted in the hospital room, I realized that I was ready to push. I sent a ward clerk to get Richard before he drove off into the night (it was midnight now) looking for a place to buy film. My messenger caught him in time and he was on hand, an able coach, as one-half hour after we arrived at the hospital door, Rienne Frances was born. She was pink and beautiful and just what her father had expected, whereas I had been sure it was a boy all those nine months. Mothers do not always know!

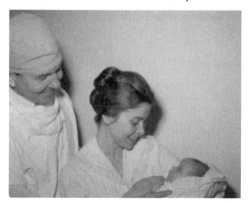

Again we enjoyed our baby at home by morning as Joey and Claryss Nan woke up. Again the baby-sitter was able to get off to school, the new baby being settled safely at home.

And again Mary Ann Kerwin delivered a huge, elegant gourmet dinner complete with birthday cake (we had enjoyed the same treat from the Kerwins for Claryss Nan's birth celebration). It is the very best birth gift you could ever give to the parents of a new baby. This idea caught on among our friends and we were all assured that food would come as a gift soon after each new baby arrived.

255

I have taken an informal survey on third babies. By and large they are the easiest to bring into the world and the hardest to fit into the family. This has nothing to do with the child, only the mothers! Often the oldest is now about four years old, still requiring help with many of the daily routines. Add to the four-year-old a two-year-old toddler who is at the most delightful stage of all (I think so anyway) but undeniably a handful, and now a brand-new baby who requires you twenty-four hours a day. You find that mothering is hard work. You now have more children than you have hands and voice commands must be obeyed. Consider the simple act of crossing the street and you see what I mean!

However, four-year-olds are becoming very "why" oriented, so a whole new world of conversing with our oldest child, Joe, was opening up. Each stage in a child's development seems more fun than the last (of course, there are also stages you can hardly wait for them to outgrow).

My theory on "stages" is that it depends upon the parents. I believe that if a parent is not threatened by a stage of development, there is no problem. If the mother or father is upset at not being obeyed, then twos are terrible. A two-year-old is testing and exploring everything—even your instructions and commands. I love the "terrible twos"! They aren't terrible at all, but challenging and exciting.

We had become a little cramped in our house by now and talked of finding a larger one. To hear Richard tell the story, it was all my idea. He says, "We were at a party one evening and I heard my wife announce that we'd be moving soon." Anyway, Rienne's first year included lots of house hunting and she grew to hate riding in a car, which our other two loved. It was one of my many "standards" about children that I had to change. By the time you've a family of three, every rule, pronouncement, generality, and prejudice that you've collected about children and parenting has been broken. We knew so much about raising children before we had any!

As Rienne was nearing her first birthday, we moved into a house with four bedrooms, one for us and one for each child. You know what happened. Our 97-percent-sure birth control put us in the other 3 percent!

Allison Lucille

Amazingly enough, my fourth pregnancy was easier than the third had been. I did not have so much pressure and thankfully I did not have so much heartburn. We were tied down to a routine now, with Joe in kindergarten and the car pool that went with it. I was very involved in baby business, teaching childbirth classes and leading La Leche League meetings. The nine months went by very quickly.

One early afternoon in April, I began to feel contractions which were regular but not too strong. I expected false labor by my fourth pregnancy and did not get too excited. It seemed a good idea to alert Richard that he might need to come home. So I called the office and told him that I was having light contractions and although they were less than ten minutes apart, I did not think it was time to go to the hospital. I'd call him when I wanted him home. He came home immediately.

By about 5 P.M. I gave in and we went to the hospital, to have the doctor tell us that although I was dilating, we could go home if we wanted until the labor picked up. We didn't want! Instead we took a "leave" from the hospital to go out for dinner. We went to a drive-in and I tried to avoid fried, greasy food. That's not easy. What I wanted was a soft-boiled egg and toast but I made do with a milk shake and hamburger. We took a drive over what seemed to be the bumpiest roads ever (every road is bumpy when you are in labor). I was ready to do anything to avoid going home to the family without a baby! We returned to the hospital and walked the halls awhile until finally my contractions increased in intensity. They had been rather close together all along—about

257

four to five minutes apart. From about midnight on I was in good, effective labor. The rest of the labor could probably be considered "false," but that's an objective decision. It seemed true when I was in it! (a 12 hour labor is not that long!)

Allison Lucille was born at 5:08 A.M., April 27. She picked a great time of day to arrive because the pediatrician made his hospital rounds by 7 A.M. He checked her and we were able to go home in our customary two hours.

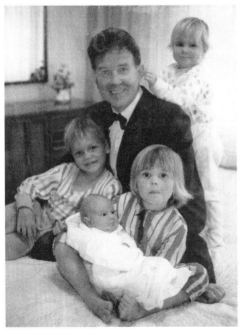

Our friends tell this story about that morning. They phoned our house to find out how things were going and when I answered the phone they assumed that I'd been in false labor and had come home empty-handed. As Florence, a mother of five, was sympathizing with my having had to go through all that false labor, I interrupted her to tell her we were home with a baby. There was dead silence on the telephone. She never got over my coming home with a two-hour-old baby! She sent over a beautiful dinner of fried chicken, though. Mary Ann brought her traditional dinner, too, another day. We ate well with new little Allison!

Although I felt great, my need to show off had subsided. I enjoyed being at home with my new baby and my little family. I hated to answer the phone. I just wanted to be alone and snuggle my baby girl. There is something so special about those first few days with a newborn.

In a very short time, however, my idyll was over and it was back to car-pooling for kindergarten, and shopping for groceries.

Allison taught me some new lessons in baby care. For one thing, a nice plump baby (eight pounds two ounces at birth) may want to change her growth patterns. The doctor ran all sorts of tests to check her health when she refused to gain weight. We both finally concluded that she was O.K. and we'd let her be the boss. She was one year old when she finally doubled her birth weight. (Most babies double by four to six months.) Bless Dr. Mijer for not being upset. Thank goodness she was our fourth and I'd already proved myself an able breastfeeding mother. Allison is still very slight though rather tall. She resists food unless it's her idea. It will help you as parents if you can accept that a baby comes to you with many individual personality traits already built in. Do not expect to "create" your child's personality. Just help it to flower and grow in the most positive way you can. I try to remember what our child psychologist friend Katherine Tennes says, "Parents take either too much credit or too much blame for their children."

Richard Evans

With our fourth pregnancy most of our friends at least tried to be politely pleased, but honestly, with the fifth there was general disapproval. My parents felt that I had enough to do and Dad had been telling us for two pregnancies to name the baby "Sufficient." Nevertheless, we all looked forward to another baby. It becomes an addiction!

Since our due date for this baby was January 5, my parents decided to come for Christmas, from their home in Parkland, Alberta, and stay till the birth. We were delighted to finally share this experience with these grandparents. Grandmother Hartman had celebrated new babies with us three times. My father always complained that Ritchie tricked us by delaying his birth ten days. Dad was anxious to get home!

This time I experienced false labor for sure. It is typical of "grand multips," as the mothers of several children are called. (Some, however, have babies more easily each time.) For three days and nights I had contractions twenty minutes apart. It was not uncomfortable but so discouraging! Richard and I went to a movie to pass the time; we went to a church annual meeting (where all the older ladies wanted to get me to the hospital immediately.) Of course, I went to the doctor. His advice was go to bed and rest. Not a bad call right after Christmas and New Years with four other children!

Finally the contractions picked up to a ten-minute interval. We checked into the hospital at 10 P.M.—fairly sure that the contractions would keep going this time. By about 3 A.M., I must have been in transition stage of labor, because though both Richard and the doctor were sleeping, I demanded their presence. The nurse didn't question my motives and called them. They dutifully sat with me for more than an hour of labor. Richard was suffering with a rather bad cold and had been doing a good coaching job for three days. Until my "witchy" transition personality, I had been perfectly content to let him rest. I was pretty good at this by now!

At last my labor moved into the pushing stage and shortly thereafter our second son was born. Again my guess had been wrong and Richard's right. It was delightful to have another boy to even up our family a bit but it made the bedroom arrangement very complicated. (We have since remodeled.)

Richard Evans Hartman checked in on January 15, and when we took him home a few hours later, there was quite a welcoming committee. Two-year-old Allison was beside herself with ecstasy. Rienne was celebrating her fourth birthday and what little girl ever had a better birthday present? The grandparents were thrilled and incredulous at both their new grandchild and their own daughter, who could enjoy the birth of her baby and be home showing him off in two hours. Joe and Claryss Nan were old hands at this experience by now, but loved it all. To Allison, it was as exciting as a new puppy as you see in the photo taken as we got home in two hours.

This child rides with the waves created by everyone else in the family. He has to! He can sit in the middle of the biggest hubbub and quietly play his own game.

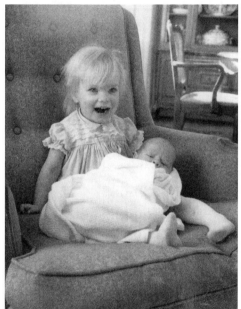

There is something special about the last baby, as you try to appreciate everything to the fullest. As with my first, I have had two years "alone" with the last. As Allison went off to school, Ritchie and I had time together. So the attention he missed as the number five child has been made up for now. The children give each other a great deal of attention, too, although some of that attention is not of a very positive variety!

It's an exciting household we have and I feel fortunate to have our large family. We are also fortunate to have "discovered" natural childbirth and to have celebrated each birth. We are indeed blessed.

Reflections

Years have passed since writing these birth stories and indeed I have been blessed.

Giving each of our children the best possible birth has given them a huge advantage in life. Natural Childbirth has enriched their lives and mine. I can't measure it, but I know that being born without drugs is a definite benefit.

My five are all grown and my darling daughters and sons and their spouses have given me nine amazing grandchildren. I have a fascinating life visiting and sharing with the next generation of this family. I am experiencing the circle of life and it is wonderful. May you have these blessings as you raise your family and bring on the next generation.

From Richard, as the Husband-Coach

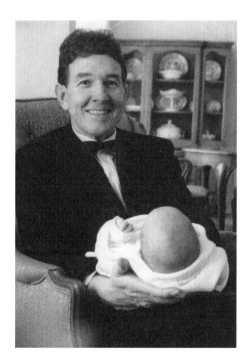

It has been a few years since my darling husband, partner, coach, best friend and soul mate died. Our years together during five pregnancies, five births and raising five children (who have become the parents of nine grandchildren for us) would not have been the success and delight it has been without Richard's enthusiastic support. My wish for you is that you have the same support from your coach or partner in your childbirth experience and in your life. With love, I will share the preface he wrote for my first book.

"I t's a boy, it's a boy, a boy, a boy, a boy!" I was shouting while jumping ten feet off the floor as our first-born, Joe, arrived—the culmination of nine months of eager anticipation.

I've been asked many times if the husband could possibly be as excited over Natural Childbirth as is his wife.

The word is: I still jump ten feet in the air at the memory of coaching my fantastically wonderful wife through five magnificent experiences resulting in five beautiful children.

Had it not been for Rhondda, I would have been gypped out of these powerful experiences, isolated in some lonely room out of communication, with suspicions that the worst was about to happen. As a matter of fact, I had given it little thought until Rhondda began educating me. Fortunately, Drs. Robert A. Bradley and Max D. Bartlett were pioneering in Natural Childbirth in my hometown, Denver. From the three of them I soon learned that a prospective father is important.

With the ultimate goal of a beautiful, healthy child in mind, I found that I could inspire my wife to train as an athlete and, with a little imagination, encourage her to exercise, eat a healthy diet, and even help make her minor discomforts more tolerable. It made sense to me that since all great athletes—from Olympic skiers to competitive horseshoe players—need coaching to perfect their skill, and since developing and having a baby is essentially physical, a coach is indeed important. I found coaching especially valuable during the tiring long labor with our first child. Rhondda needed my constant chatter of: "Come on, Rhondda baby, relax"—"Float this one out"—"Gee, that's really great"—"I'm really proud of you"—"This has been going on for hours and you've been riding them out like a dream"—"You keep this up and you'll be writing a book"—"O.K., you're probably getting close to transition"—"This is going to be a little tough, but relax because you're about to push"—"You can ride it out—remember, this time it's a short one"—"Aren't you getting excited?"—"Hey, nurse, check this one's dilation—she's about to go to press!"

I have to confess that during those wee hours of the night I had a tendency to put my head down and fall asleep, under the impression that Rhondda really didn't need me. She corrected me later. My best efforts were most helpful and most needed as Rhondda reached transition—those last contractions before pushing begins. The most exciting time for both of us was the pushing. I found the participation in the miracle of birth and the anticipation of seeing my own child come into the world superlative and exhilarating. When the final moment of truth did come, I feel convinced I really did jump ten feet off the floor out of sheer pent-up excitement.

Richard E. Hartman

This is an actual letter written to my only sister, Clarice Evans Siebens, and her husband, Bill, in Calgary, Alberta, when they were expecting their first child, Carter. They now have two more, Rhondda and Evann. They also have eight grandchildren! The doctor was helpful and the birth experiences were happy. I include it because it was the actual beginning of this book ... and because she is my beloved only sister.

Please read it as a capsule in time from when we began to have husbands in the birthing room! It shows that what I was teaching then has not really changed from what Natural Childbirth is today. Natural doesn't change!

Dear Clarice & Bill,

How I wish you could be here to have your baby with us where we have classes, sympathetic doctors, and a hospital that allows couples to stay together for a birth. Naturally, you are concerned. Childbirth is

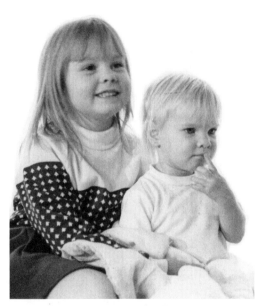

Claryss Nan and Allison ...
Next Generation Sisters

such an "unknown" with your first baby. Read the books I've recommended. Remember the talks we've had about my childbirth experiences. Now, here are some last-minute reminders to help you be ready for the most exciting thing that will ever happen to you both.

For pregnancy and back comfort, the pelvic rock is best. Standing posture is extremely important—hold your pelvis level rather than letting the baby's weight pull your tummy out and your back into a sway. Do eighty pelvic rocks on all fours just before bed *every* night. No matter how tired you are, do those bedtime pelvic rocks! It is easy enough to work in the other pelvic rocks when it's convenient during the day.

Get off your feet and put them up as often as possible even though you may not feel the need. Varicose veins run in our family, and it's almost a normal thing with pregnancy.

For labor, become proficient at abdominal breathing and relaxing. These may take a great deal of control and effort as your labor progresses, so practice as soon as you feel contractions—even though not hard ones—so you'll be an old hand at it by late first stage. This is all you do throughout your whole first-stage labor—relax and tummy-breathe with each contraction. Be sure to breathe out as completely as in to prevent hyperventilation, which makes your fingers get stiff during labor and is easily cured by breathing into a paper bag, or cupped hands, so you breathe some carbon dioxide.

We find that the time for the most control on your part is transition, or when the cervix is seven to ten centimeters dilated. Carry on with abdominal breathing and *complete* relaxation. Here it helps if you have something to think about, for example, the picture a friend painted for me of the clouds or the view from Jungfrau Joch—these are what I used—as well as Richard's reassurance and encouragement: "You are doing fine, things are going well, let yourself relax," etc. This transition is a relatively short time in labor—trickiest but shortest!

Second stage is pushing and you have no choice in the matter. Your body lets you do *nothing* else, so don't resist but work with it. It's automatic and it's marvelous. This is where you will be expected to "take something" and this is where the fun comes in. You work hard but if you will raise your head, as though trying to see the baby coming, and push hard enough, you will have no pain—honest. This does not require any "control," only hard pushing such as you'd do with a very constipated bowel movement, only harder work. (I hate to say that except it is one way for you to know *how* to push!) Take a deep breath and hold it while you push. Let it out in a gush when you can't hold your breath any longer, take another big chest breath, and keep pushing as long as there is any contraction. The doctor may have to tell you when to stop pushing, as sometimes it's not definite to you but he can see when the contraction is over.

Plead with your doctor to read Dr. Bradley's book so that his help can be more than to "offer you something." What you'll need is encouragement, *not* gas or drugs or an epidural, so that you can be awake to push and for the excitement of the birth!

In case your doctor asks you: yes, we do episiotomies, and the pressure of crowning and pushing makes its own natural anesthetic for the cutting (midline usually, if possible), but a local is given for suturing after the birth of the baby.

Richard's word for Bill: do not worry if labor is long. It can go on for hours and hours and be very normal. Apparently he became worried with Joey, as it took fifteen hours all told—but I was too busy relaxing and enjoying a new experience to realize he was worried, and he, bless him, did not tell me! The advantage of a long labor is that you get good at everything as you go along! *Expect* it to be long, then you'll not be disappointed. (Fifteen hours is not long, but it is with Natural Childbirth.)

Gosh, I wish I could talk with you. I'm not trying to *tell* you what to do unless this is what you want in the first place. Anything that makes your experiences in childbirth happy and pleasant cannot be failure, no matter how far you go with our methods. I am convinced that a happy labor changes your general attitude to the children and your husband.

Another point—when you are pushing, you look as though you are in pain. The picture of me pushing makes everyone feel sympathy, and maybe this is why they shove gas at you. Of course, it hurts if you don't push!

Never, never, never lie flat on your back during labor. They may do your "prep" and leave you lying that way. Either roll over on your side with leg drawn up and arm behind you or in a contour, half-sitting/ half-lying position on your back (hospital beds crank into this position at knee and back), with pillows under your arms or wherever needed to help you be comfy. Change position when you get stiff or uncomfortable. Move about in between contractions, especially until transition.

Rienne cut her "right front top center" tooth today and is a bit fussy. She's so funny—all teeth (seven)—much like Joey as a baby with more hair—not long hair, but really thick.

The other two are sweet as ever. Joey has come out of his "frightful four" stage and is a darling again. Claryss Nan is amazing—we were withholding dessert because she had not eaten her main course, so she rushed off and brought Richard's slippers and put them on. Naturally, she got dessert! She seems to understand the power of a smile, and really throws on the charm!

One more word on Natural Childbirth before I mail this:

 It's good for Uncle Bill to know that having a baby requires, more or less, the same amount of energy needed to play four quarters of football—hence the necessity of preparing by exercising in advance. Also, this amount of work, with no half-time break, requires lots of encouragement and help from the coach—namely Bill. He'll be able to stay with you till nearly pushing time probably—and it will be a marvelous help. It's ghastly to be left alone during labor and nurses are usually too busy—and it's dull for them! The only one you'll really want is Bill anyway. At first you can play cards or visit, but later you'll just need to know he's there. Bill —I'm writing this for you. Never will you be more proud of and proud to be with Clarice—so be a good papa. Hold her hand but be firm about her relaxing and tummy breathing. It could be a long time.

Remember, you would be perfect at this if you had perfect circumstances. Any amount of comfort and enjoyment you gain from all this is worth it and if you do things differently from us, that's O.K. It's a glorious experience and it's the end result that's best of all! (Writing this all down makes me ready to have another.)

Love and kisses,
Your big sis,
Rhondda

$\big\{$ ACKNOWLEDGMENTS

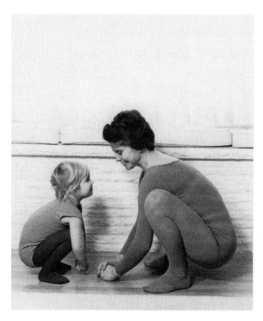

Rienne with me in a Squat

My Artist – Deborah Springer and I have been friends since our children were babies. She and her husband Charles came to my classes with three of their four births. We became La Leche League Leaders together and have stayed friends. She has believed in me and has kept these sketches for years waiting for me to get this book in print. They live in Boulder, Colorado and Debbie now draws and paints there, and around the world in their RV and during their sailing trips. She is a grandmother to "Rhondda's Babies" since her daughters used my book with their pregnancies and births. Thank you, Debbie.

My Book Shepherd – One wonders if this book would ever have happened had it not been for my meeting of Judith Briles, whirling wonder woman of the publishing world. I met her by phone through Colorado Authors' League. She invited me to the first AuthorU meeting, I went, was impressed, kept going and now I have learned enough and been coddled and supported enough by Judith that here I am … an author again!

I am honored to be in Judith's embrace. She is an amazing mentor and friend and also my slave driver. She is a human dynamo who has never been confronted by a job too large. Impossible is not in her vocabulary. I could not have done it without her. I did not get it done until I found her! Thank you, Judith.

My Editor and Indexer – John Maling, editor extraordinaire, has a library of knowledge in his head as he sits faithfully over a manuscript that once again has new material for him to absorb and make readable. He moves phrases around and turns mundane writing into literature, well, that is not always possible but he improves a writer's image every time. Mine included. Thank you, John.

My Book Designer – Nick Zelinger's creative genius brings vision and flexibility to my book. He brings life to Debbie's wonderful illustrations and makes my words interesting, easy to read and a veritable visual feast. His flexibility and ideas on presentation made such a difference. Thank you, Nick.

The Bradley Method® – There would be no modern teaching of The Bradley Method® without Marjie and Jay Hathaway. Dr. Bradley saw in them the passion to keep his legacy alive and he was so right. They have been true to his passion and have made sure it survived another generation as their son James has taken over much of the business and their daughter Susan has been a devoted educator and writer to support the Academy of Husband Coached Childbirth. Marjie has given me huge encouragement with her time, updating and validating the need for me to get this book finished. I appreciate the enthusiasm and support from the The Bradley Method®. Thank you, Hathaways.

My Friend Susan – When Dr. Bradley married his beloved Martha, she brought with her a sweet daughter who did not want to move to Denver! That teenager has matured, is the lovely mother of twins, managed Dr. Bradley's busy office and has become one of my very dear friends, Susan Nelson. She and her sisters, Martha and Maryann hold the copyright to the book, *Husband Coached Childbirth* written by Dr. Bradley and which has been revised by the Hathaways. The book is the centerpiece of The Bradley Method. The three sisters have supported and encouraged me in a way that makes me feel as though Dr. Bradley is with us still. Martha, a beautiful petite lady whose soft Southern drawl masked a sterling strong woman, was also my dear friend and I miss her. Thank you to the three Bradley daughters who are in my corner always. Thank you, Susan.

Doctor Bradley – And then there is the good doctor who had a passion and an urgency to save babies from the harm of obstetrical drugs which were the standard of care. He is also the first to have husbands be with their wives during the birth. He never saw a hurdle he could not climb over or knock down. He was a huge man with a very strong personality that could encompass a stadium. One could say the man had a very large aura! He took on negativity as a challenge. He told his story of babies being drugged at birth where ever he saw an audience. He had a reputation among radio and TV interviewers that once Dr. Bradley got the microphone you could never get it back! He spoke quickly and with conviction. He thrived on controversy. He knew he was right about fathers at the birth. He knew drugs were harmful to babies. He did not listen to the standards set by his profession. They were wrong. He never stopped fighting for babies to be born drug free and into the welcoming arms of a mother who gave birth naturally and would breastfeed her baby. Honestly, the man was a force of nature to be reckoned with. It has been my honor to know him, to be his friend and to have worked with him in his relentless cause for mothers and babies.

My Family – How do I properly thank my family? What would my life be without them? It is my life and my love. It is fun and heart ache. It is pride and joy, embarrassment and anger. It is life to the fullest. Mothering encompasses it all. Life has no meaning for me without my family. They are my best support and my best critics. I am alternately the best and the worst. I am to blame and I made it happen. Let us face it … I am a mother. I am Unconditional Love. I am where the buck stops. I am the go to person. I've even been called in the middle of the night to give permission to go to the hospital, for heaven's sake! I've been accused of giving birth to them so I could write a book! So, Thanks, kids, for giving me enough to write about! Twice!!

My Photographers –

Nicholas De Scoise

Gene Hinrichs

They each took photographs in my eighth and ninth months of my last two pregnancies. I used their photos in my first book and now some of them have been used herein. You will recognize them as artistic family photos! Thank you.

My Videographer – Evann Siebens is my niece. In her ninth month at a family Christmas visit, we managed to do a shoot with her multitasking as the model, director and videographer. We had a lot of fun doing it and amazingly, I think you will find it very helpful and explanatory as well as fun. It is as close as I could come to being right there with you teaching the exercises. She is the wonderful mother of two beautiful children now and I hope she will find time to give you the advantage of an instructional DVD to compliment this book. She is a busy documentary film producer as well as having several Art Installations to her credit in museums in the United States, England and Canada. Thanks, Evann.

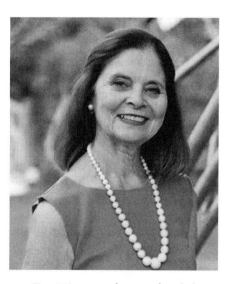

Rhondda Evans Hartman grew up in southern Alberta, Canada where she was a Public Health Nurse before becoming a homemaker and mother. She moved to Colorado after marrying Denver Attorney, Richard E. Hartman in Switzerland while vacationing in Europe. They created five amazing children who have produced nine incredible grandchildren.

She earned her B.S. from the University of Alberta, where she was Vice President of the Student Council in her senior year. She completed her R.N. at the University of Alberta Hospital, School of Nursing in Edmonton, Alberta and became the Public Health Nurse in Lacombe, Alberta. Many years later after all her children were in school, she earned a Master of Arts Degree in Urban Sociology from the University of Colorado in Denver.

For 25 years, she taught classes and trained and supervised other teachers in husband-coached childbirth for Dr. Robert A. Bradley in his Obstetrical Medical Practice in Denver, Colorado. Rhondda is on the Advisory Board of the American Academy of Husband Coached Childbirth, The Bradley Method. She is Charter Member and past president of La Leche League of Colorado and was a meeting leader for many years. Rhondda and Dr. Bradley were frequent speakers at national Natural Childbirth conferences. As an expert on Natural Childbirth exercises, she personally has instructed over 14,000 mothers in having a natural and enjoyable birth. Rhondda has been a guest on national TV in both the United States and Canada.

Natural Childbirth Exercises is her second book. She is also the author of *Exercises for True Natural Childbirth* and is a contributor to the *Five Standards for Safe Childbearing* by David Stewart, PhD. and *Compulsory Hospitalization or Freedom of Choice in Childbirth?* by Stewart and Stewart, editors.

Contact Rhondda through her website:

www.NaturalChildbirthExercises.com

Follow Rhondda and Natural Childbirth Exercises on:
Twitter: @BirthExercises
Facebook: NationalChildbirthExercises
Pinterest: Natural Childbirth Exercises – Rhondda Hartman
Blog: http://NaturalChildbirthExercises.com/blog
LinkedIn Group: Natural Childbirth Exercises

bowel 73, 76, 148, 183

Bradley, Dr. Robert A. 1, 4-8, 11-12, 33, 38, 45, 50, 64, 121, 134, 151, 190, 237, 245, 253, 264, 274-5, 277

Bradley Method Class 10, 82-3, 221

breastfeeding (*see also* feeding) 97, 127-41, 143-5, 169, 207, 213, 227, 229, 239, 253, 259

  folklore 129

  mothers 129, 132, 138, 213, 231

breasts 13, 42, 52, 81, 127-8, 132-3, 135-7, 139-40, 144-5, 163-4, 187, 203-4, 206, 212

breath 15, 61-5, 118-19, 121-4, 126, 141, 147-8, 170, 190, 193, 195-6, 249, 269

breathe 56, 58, 61-5, 120, 123, 165, 170, 174, 179, 212, 249, 268

breathing 53, 61-5, 110, 118, 120, 123, 171, 175-6, 180, 191, 207, 268

breech 209-11

buttocks 36, 42-4, 47, 77, 234

C

calm 59, 136, 190, 192, 219, 248-9

calories 94-6

carbohydrates 91-2, 94-6, 101

centimeters (*see also* dilation) 172-4, 179, 268

cervix 123, 167, 171-4, 179, 189, 268

chest 29, 39, 52, 56, 64, 68, 111, 120-2, 140, 147-8, 164, 170, 193-5, 249-50

  muscles 139, 141

childbirth 3, 5-6, 11-12, 18, 21, 50, 77, 82, 158, 267, 270, 278

  coached 274, 277

  educated 19, 82

  educator 3, 130, 239, 253

  experiences 16, 21, 49, 244, 263, 268

circulation 27, 33-5, 41, 45, 62, 104, 106, 110, 112, 114, 140, 174, 226

clothes 42, 68, 144, 149

coach 20, 26, 53-4, 64, 125-6, 147-8, 171, 175-6, 180, 184-5, 190, 194-6, 207, 209, 238, 246-7, 263-4

coaching 123, 147, 180, 183, 190, 195-6, 264

colostrum 135-6

contour position 52, 62-3, 65, 125

contractions 49-51, 54, 58-65, 119, 122-3, 134-5, 159-62, 168-71, 174-6, 179-82, 185, 192-4, 201-2, 248-51, 260, 268-70

cord, umbilical 164, 198, 203

couples 5-6, 8, 153, 158, 213, 216, 246-7, 267

crying baby (*see also* baby, crying) 136, 217-20, 225

cystocele 76

D

delivery 8, 74-5, 163, 209-10, 231, 250

diet 85, 87-8, 91-4, 96-9, 100-2, 106, 128, 131-2, 160, 205, 239, 255, 259, 264

digestive system 85-6

V

W

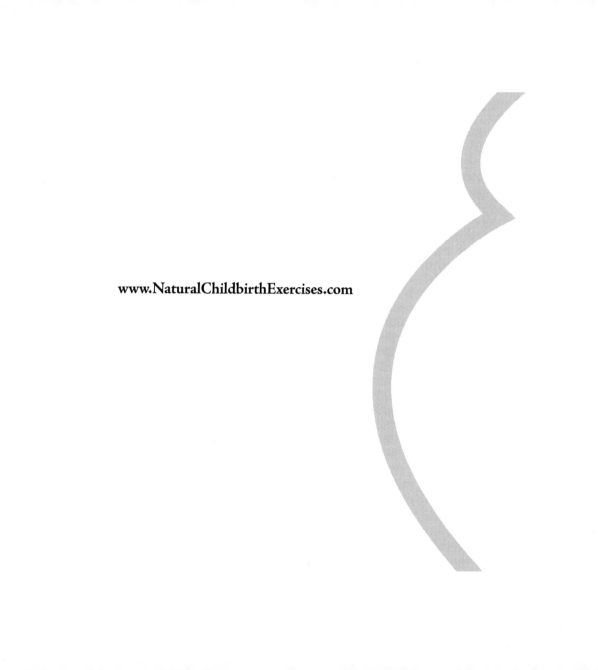

www.NaturalChildbirthExercises.com